Fundamentals of Clinical Ophthalmology

Neuro-ophthalmology

For Hazel

Fundamentals of Clinical Ophthalmology

Neuro-ophthalmology

James Acheson

Consultant Ophthalmologist, National Hospital for Neurology and Neurosurgery, London, UK

Paul Riordan-Eva

Consultant Ophthalmologist, King's College Hospital, London, UK

Series Editor:

Susan Lightman

Professor of Clinical Ophthalmology, Institute of Ophthalmology/Moorfields Eye Hospital, London, UK

© BMJ Books 1999
BMJ Books is an imprint of the BMJ Publishing Group

First published in 1999
by BMJ Books, BMA House, Tavistock Square,
London WC1H 9JR

British Library Cataloguing in Publication Data

A catalogue record for this book is available from the
British Library

ISBN 0-7279-1369-7

Typeset, printed and bound in Great Britain by
Latimer Trend & Company Ltd, Plymouth

Contents

Contributors

James F Acheson
Consultant Ophthalmologist, National Hospital for Neurology and Neurosurgery

FD Bremner
Research Fellow, Department of Neuro-Ophthalmology, National Hospital for Neurology and Neurosurgery

Lorraine Cassidy
Clinical Fellow, Department of Neuro-Ophthalmology, National Hospital for Neurology and Neurosurgery

Peter J Goadsby
Professor and Consultant Neurologist, Institute of Neurology and National Hospital for Neurology and Neurosurgery

Tim Mathews
Research Fellow, Department of Neuro-Ophthalmology, National Hospital for Neurology and Neurosurgery

Preface

To limit ophthalmology to the study of the eye and peripheral processes of vision is to mutilate unreasonably the most comprehensive subject in the whole of medicine.

SIR STUART DUKE ELDER, 1949

Neuro-ophthalmology is one of the bonds which joins ophthalmology to medicine and neuroscience and opens up a wider world of visual disorders. It encompasses a range of topics incorporating the neurobiology of vision and large portions of clinical neurology and clinical ophthalmology. In addition, there are overlaps with neuroradiology, neurosurgery, and neurophysiology as well as radiotherapy, neuro-otology, and head and neck surgery. The trainee ophthalmologist is led a long way from the familiar challenges of surgical problems of the globe and orbit and has to learn how to apply ophthalmic clinical methods to the solution of visual problems arising from within the brain. Hopefully in some small way this basic text can help ophthalmologists to start to feel at home in this territory and to realise how important a basic knowledge of the subject material is to the everyday care of patients with all the multitude of visual problems with which they may present.

James Acheson and Paul Riordan-Eva

Acknowledgements

Permission to reproduce the following illustrations is gratefully acknowledged:

Figure 0.1 is reproduced from MacLaren RE, Regeneration and transplantation in the optic nerve: developing a clinical strategy, *Br J Ophthalmol* 1998;**82**:577–84.

Figure 1.1 is reproduced from Acheson JF and Sanders MD. *Common problems in neuro-ophthalmology*. London: WB Saunders, 1997. Figure 1.2 is reproduced from Lee WR. *Ophthalmic histopathology*. Berlin: Springer-Verlag, 1993. Figure 1.3 is reproduced from Olver JM, Spalton DJ, McCartney AC. Quantitative morphology of human retrolaminar optic nerve vasculature. *Invest Ophthalmol Vis Sci* 1994;**35**(11):3858–66. Figure 1.4 is after Glaser JS. *Neuro-ophthalmology*, 2nd edn. Philadelphia: Lippincott, 1990. Figure 1.5 is reproduced from Gross CG. *Brain, vision and memory – tales in the history of neuroscience*. Boston, MA: MIT Press, 1998:66. Figure 1.6 is reproduced from Polyak S. *The vertebrate visual system*. Chicago: Chicago University Press, 1957. Figure 1.7 is reproduced from Zeki S. *A vision of the brain*. Oxford: Blackwell, 1993. Figure 1.8 is after Mishkin M, Ungerlieder LG, Macko K. Object vision and spatial vision: two cortical pathways. *Trends Neurosci* 1983;**6**:414–17.

Figure 2.2(a) is copyright of Steven Newman and is reproduced with permission from Feldon SE. Visual fields in retinal disease. In: Ryan SJ (ed.) *Retina*, vol. 1, ch. 13. St Louis: Mosby, 1989. Figure 2.2(b) is after Anderson DR. *Testing the field of vision*. St Louis: Mosby, 1982. Figures 2.8 and 2.9 are reproduced from Holder GE. *J Neurol Neurosurg Psychiatry* 1989;**52**:1364–9.

Figure 4.1(c) is reproduced from Corbett JJ, Savino PJ, Thompson HS *et al. Arch Neurol* 1982;**39**:461–74.

Figures 6.2 and 6.4 are reproduced from Slamovits TL, Burde R. *Neuro-ophthalmology*. St Louis: Mosby, 1994.

Figure 10.2 is reproduced from Rosen ES, Thompson HS, Cumming WJ, Eustace P. *Neuro-ophthalmology*. London: Mosby, 1997.

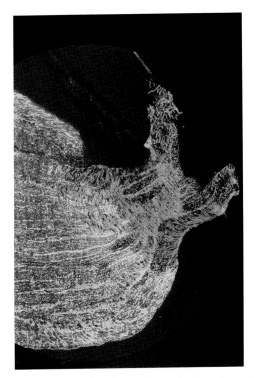

Figure 0.1   The glial interface at the retina–optic nerve junction. Astrocytes of the lamina cribrosa and nerve fibre layer of the retina are labelled with antibodies to glial fibrillary acidic protein (green). Oligodendrocytes of the optic nerve are labelled with antibodies to myelin basic protein (orange). The dense myelin in this region needs to be neutralised or bypassed for optic nerve regeneration to be successful. (Reproduced with permission from MacLaren RE, Regeneration and transplantation in the optic nerve: developing a clinical strategy. Br J Ophthalmol *1998;82:577–84)*

1: Synopsis of anatomy and physiology of the visual sensory system

JF ACHESON

1.1 The organisation of the human visual sensory system – parallel processing and retinotopy

Retinotopy

The retinal ganglion cells project to the brain according to the principle of retinotopy. This refers to the fact that the point-by-point correspondence of the representation of visual space on the retina is preserved in the visual pathways all the way from each eye to both cortical hemispheres. In this way the superior visual field is transmitted by the inferior retina and is mediated by inferior axons in the optic nerve, chiasm, optic tract, radiations, and cortex. At the chiasm, fibres from the ganglion cells nasal to the fovea cross to merge with non-crossing fibres from the temporal retina of the contralateral eye. As a result, fibres from each eye representing common points in the visual field come to be aligned together in the optic tract. The precision of this alignment increases towards the cortex, while in the lateral geniculate ganglion the retinotopic map is rotated through 90 degrees. The interpretation of visual field defects rests heavily on an appreciation of the principle of

1

retinotopy, for example when we try to determine whether a patient with bilateral visual failure has a problem in the anterior or the posterior (post-chiasmal) visual pathways.

Parallel processing

Distinct classes of neurones process visual information from retina to cortex in parallel streams; those primarily dealing with colour vision, high spatial resolution, and fine static stereopsis are referred to as parvocellular (referring to the relatively small size of the cell bodies and axons of one subpopulation of retinal ganglion cells – P cells) and those dealing primarily with motion detection, low spatial resolution, and coarse motion stereopsis are referred to as magnocellular (retinal ganglion cells with larger cells bodies and coarser calibre axons – M cells). P cells make up around 80% of the retinal ganglion cells (RGCs), M cells 10%, and the remainder are cells which have midbrain projections.[1] Parvocellular and magnocellular neurones are also morphologically distinct in the lateral geniculate ganglion and cortex, and further subsystems may also exist. The parvocellular stream can be further segregated into two substreams, parvo-blob and parvo-interblob. Blobs are clusters of cells in the primary visual cortex that stain intensely for cytochrome oxidase indicating high metabolic activity. The parvo-interblob stream appears to be involved with fine spatial acuity and the parvo-blob in colour discrimination. Although these parallel streams characterise the organisation of the visual system, the picture is complicated by the fact that there are extensive interactions between the subsystems at a cortical level and oversimplification may be misleading.[2,3] None the less, an appreciation of these arrangements is helpful in the understanding of a variety of pathological processes including cerebral achromatopsia, motion blindness, blindsight, and stato-kinetic dissociation (see below).

1.2   The anterior visual pathways: retina, optic nerve, and chiasm

Retina

The retina contains the initial neural substrate for the transmission of visual information from the eye to the cortex. Vision in

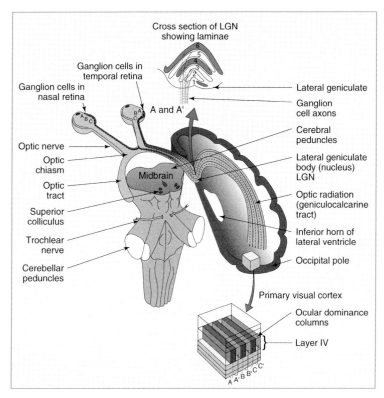

Figure 1.1   Overall scheme of the visual pathways. The manner of retinotopic projection to the lateral geniculate ganglion (LGN) and the ocular dominance columns in the primary visual cortex from left and right eyes is illustrated by three imaginary points or images (A, B,C) from the left visual field (not shown) falling on the right half of each retina (A,B, C in the left eye and A', B', C' in the right eye).

the retina is served at three neuronal levels: the photoreceptor, the bipolar cell, and the ganglion cell, which projects to the lateral geniculate ganglion.

During embryogenesis the inner layer of the invaginated optic vesicle differentiates to form the layers of the neurosensory retina – the photoreceptors, the outer nuclear and outer plexiform layers, the inner nuclear and inner plexiform layers, the ganglion cell layer, and the nerve fibre layer (from choroid to vitreous). Müller (glial) cells extend vertically through the whole thickness of the retina. The high concentration of ganglion cells around the posterior pole leads to a layer four to six cells thick surrounding the fovea, but high resolution acuity at the fovea itself is facilitated by the displacement of all retinal elements aside, allowing light energy to reach the photoreceptors directly. The neurosensory retina is hierarchically organised into vertical networks in which first order cells are connected to a smaller number of second order cells and second order cells connected to a smaller number of third order cells. There are around three retinal ganglion cells (RGCs) per foveal cone and between the central and peripheral retina RGC density changes by a factor of 1–4000.[4]

Blood supply of the retina

The main branches of the central retinal artery and vein traverse the retina at the level of the inner plexiform layer – capillaries penetrate as deep as the inner nuclear layer only, and cells of the bipolar, outer plexiform, outer nuclear, and photoreceptor layers are supplied from the choroid. Where the retinal nerve fibre layer is thickest, in the arcuate bundles and in the peripapillary area, an extra layer of capillaries is found. The retinal blood vessels have autoregulatory properties capable of functioning without neural control. An increased pressure gradient across the vessel wall produced by a rise in intraluminal pressure or a fall in intraocular pressure results in vasoconstriction both in arteries and veins.

Optic nerve

Functionally, the optic nerve begins with the ganglion cells of the retina. RGCs more peripherally located in the retina project to the periphery of the optic nerve head and are also located more deeply in the nerve fibre layers as they approach the disc. Peripapillary ganglion cells project to the centre of the optic nerve.

Axons from ganglion cells in the macula area around the fovea form a spindle shaped maculopapillar bundle which enters the optic nerve head on the temporal side. Fibres from the remaining retina take an arcuate course to reach the optic nerve at the superior and inferior poles. Altogether, there are about 1 million axons in each optic nerve, conducting partially processed visual information from the retinal ganglion cells to the lateral geniculate ganglion. Axons making up the centrocaecal projection (both the foveal projection and the projection of RGCs between the fovea and the

4

optic disc) travel together to the temporal optic nerve and remain substantially separate from the peripheral fibres, at least initially.[5]

The retinal nerve fibre layer in the temporal retina is divided about a horizontal raphé with axons originating from the superior retina arching over the fovea to reach the superior optic nerve head, and fibres from the inferior retina arching beneath the fovea. This division of retinal nerve fibres reflects the displacement of all retinal elements except the photoreceptors away from the fovea, and defines the horizontal meridian of the visual field throughout the visual system. As a result, ganglion cells adjacent to each other in the temporal retina send projections to remote parts of the optic nerve. Nearly a third of all axons in the optic nerve serve the central 5 degrees of field. Near the globe these are clustered in the central and temporal portion of the optic nerve (foveal projection) but more proximally they become intermingled with fibres serving peripheral vision throughout the nerve. Approaching the chiasm, fibres destined to decussate shift into progressively more nasal positions in the posterior optic nerve.

The optic nerve can conveniently be described in terms of four parts: the optic nerve head, the intraorbital optic nerve, the intraosseous (intracanalicular) optic nerve, and the intracranial optic nerve. The optic nerve head is subdivided according to its relationship with the lamina cribrosa in the scleral canal into prelaminar, laminar, and retrolaminar portions. Axons from the retinal ganglion cells exit the eye by turning 90 degrees to pass through the scleral canal and fibrous septa of the lamina cribrosa. At this point they become myelinated and the optic nerve head is formed. In some individuals the optic nerve exits the sclera at less than a 90 degree angle – as a result a halo shaped crescent of choroid and/or sclera is exposed at the nerve head margin on one side and an elevated sharply rolled disc margin is seen opposite. This tilted disc is a common normal variant. In addition to axons, the nerve head is composed of supportive astrocytes, myelin forming oligodendrocytes, and blood vessels. Capillary sized blood vessels supply the optic nerve head tissues while the central retinal artery and vein course through it. The orbital optic nerve is between 20 and 30 mm long and 3–4 mm in diameter, extending in an S-shape from the globe to the optic foramen at the orbital apex. The nerve is surrounded by pia, arachnoid, and dura – the latter layer forming in continuity with the sclera. At the apex of the orbit, elements of the dura fuse with periosteum and the origin of the extraocular muscles at the annulus of Zinn. Between 5 and 15 mm posterior to the globe the central retinal artery enters and the central retinal vein exits the nerve by the inferonasal margin. At the orbital apex the optic nerve is surrounded by the fibrous circle of Zinn – the origin of the four rectus muscles. The superior and medial recti also take origin from the nerve sheath itself – this is thought to be the explanation for the pain on eye movements which is a common symptom of inflammatory optic nerve disease.

The intraosseous/intracanalicular optic nerve passes through the optic canal – formed by the union of the two roots of the lesser wing of the sphenoid bone. Generally the canal is covered by bone and dura but the bony wall is often incomplete posterior to the foramen, particularly medially in relation to the sphenoid and posterior ethmoid sinuses. Each canal runs posteriorly and medially, transmitting the optic nerve and ophthalmic artery tethered within a dural lining.

The intracranial optic nerve extends about 10 mm (3–16 mm) medially and posteriorly and superiorly to reach the chiasm. The frontal lobe of the brain lies superiorly, the anterior cerebral and anterior communicating arteries and olfactory nerve lie medially, and the internal carotid and ophthalmic artery origin lie laterally. The sphenoid sinus lies inferiorly.

Vascular supply of the optic nerve head

At the most superficial level, the prelaminar portion of the optic nerve head derives its blood supply from direct branches of the central retinal artery. The laminar and retrolaminar portions are supplied by branches of the short posterior ciliary vessels via the anastamotic circle of Zinn–Haller. The circle of Zinn–Haller also derives input from the peripapillary choroid and the pial arterial network.[6] Although autoregulation of blood flow is thought to be absent in the choroidal circulation (and present in the retinal), the healthy optic nerve head can nevertheless maintain a steady blood flow in the face of fluctuations of intraocular and arterial perfusion pressure. These arrangements are of great clinical importance because vascular insufficiency of the optic nerve head has been implicated in the commonest optic neuropathy of all – glaucoma, as well as in acute anterior ischaemic optic neuropathy.

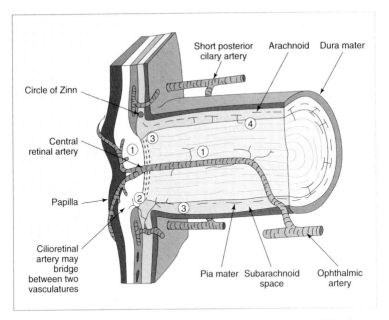

Figure 1.2   Blood supply of the optic nerve. The four sources of vessels supplying the optic nerve include: (1) branches of the central retinal artery; (2) branches from the circle of Zinn; (3) choroidal branches; (4) pial branches.

Optic chiasm

The inferior aspect of the chiasm lies about 10 mm above the plane of the diaphragma sellae, and the plane of the visual pathways at this point is inclined some 45 degrees as nerve fibres sweep backwards and upwards into the optic tracts. Lateral to the chiasm lies the supraclinoid portion of the internal carotid artery: the anterior cerebral arteries pass over the dorsal aspect of the optic nerves as they converge. It is clear therefore that intrasellar tumours such as pituitary adenomas must expand some distance in the suprasellar cistern before impinging on the visual pathways. For this reason, functioning adenomas are more likely to present to the endocrinologist and non-functioning tumours to the ophthalmologist.

At the chiasm fibres originating from ganglion cells located nasal to the fovea cross into the contralateral optic tract. Some ventral crossing fibres loop briefly into the opposite nerve before entering the tract (von Wilbrand's knee). Fibres serving the central 5 degrees

7

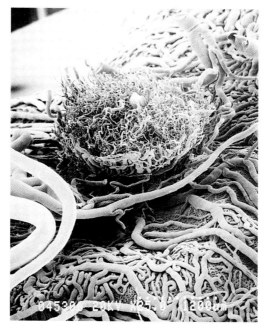

*Figure 1.3   Methylmethacrylate cast of the microvascular anatomy of the posterior ciliary
vessels, choroid and pial capillary plexus.*

(foveal projection) become dispersed in the posterior optic nerve
and are now thought to be distributed throughout the chiasm. At
the chiasm the partial decussation of optic nerve fibres merges
input from the two hemi-retinas subserving contralateral fields of
vision.

1.3   The anterior visual pathways: normal and abnormal development

The optic nerve develops from the neuroectoderm of the optic
stalk which is first apparent in the 4 mm human embryo. By the
17 mm stage the stalk has elongated with a lumen communicating
proximally with the forebrain cavity and with a distal segment
invaginated by surface ectoderm. At this stage nerve fibres begin
to grow from the ganglion cells of the retina and the embryonic
cleft begins to close. Some retinal cells become isolated at the
centre of the presumptive optic disc: these cells together with the

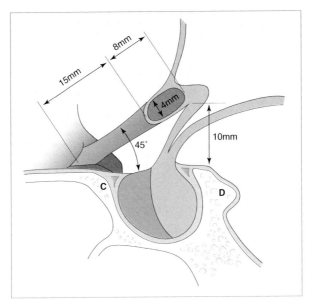

Figure 1.4 Sagittal section to show relationship between the pituitary fossa and the anterior visual pathway: note that a mass arising in the pituitary fossa usually has to extend at least 1 cm above the sella to cause any visual deficit.

hyaloid artery form the primitive epithelial papilla of Bergmeister. The lips of the distal embryonic cleft fuse to enclose the hyaloid artery, which eventually becomes the intraneural portion of the central retinal artery. After birth the intraocular hyaloid vessels disappear together with the papilla leaving the physiological optic disc cup. Entering the optic stalk, the nerve fibres of the RGCs invade the invaginating inner layer of the optic vesicle and proceed towards the brain. By the 25 mm stage the whole of the lumen has been filled with nerve fibres. The cavity of the optic vesicle no longer communicates with that of the forebrain where the site is marked by the optic recess in the floor of the third ventricle. Growing proximally to reach the optic recess, the fibres intermix to form the chiasmal decussation. The lateral geniculate body differentiates from the thalamus at the 30 mm stage and with the formation of the optic tract at 48 mm the anterior visual pathway is complete. Uncrossed fibres do not appear until the 59 mm (11th week) stage and by the 80 mm (13th week) stage the adult arrangement of partial decussation is complete. At 16–17 weeks' gestation a peak of 3.7 million axons can be identified in the optic

9

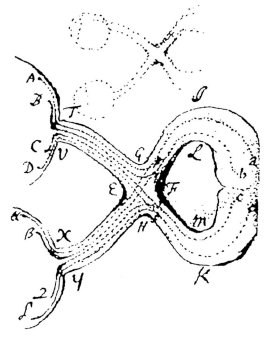

Figure 1.5 Isaac Newton was among the first to suggest in 1704 that there is a partial decussation of axons at the optic chiasm, as shown in this sketch.

nerve. This is followed by a very rapid decline to the normal adult number of 1.1 million by 31 weeks.[7]

Primitive glial cells are formed from the same multipotential cells which at a very early stage lose their bipotentiality and develop into cells which are committed to either neuronal or glial lineage. By the second half of the 2nd month a dense network of neuroglial cells has formed in the distal part of the optic nerve which are orientated perpendicularly to the nerve fibres: these constitute the first elements of the lamina cribrosa. At this stage the network is entirely comprised of type-1 astrocytes, but during the 4th month type-2 astrocytes and oligodendrocytes differentiate under the regulation of various growth factors. Malfunctions of this differentiation underlie the pathogenesis of childhood optochiasmal glioma. Surrounding mesoderm also becomes incorporated into the optic nerve to form the system of septa. By the 6th and 7th months the arachnoid sheath has differentiated between pia and dura, the pia and the arachnoid being largely of the same neuro-

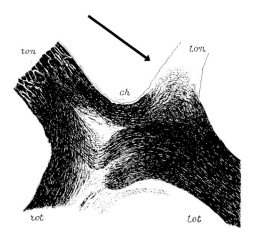

Figure 1.6   Horizontal section of the human optic chiasm stained by the Weigert method in a patient whose left eye was lost 24 years before death. The left optic nerve (lon) is completely atrophic. Fibres of the right optic nerve (ron) enter the left optic tract (lot) and right optic tract (rot). The arrow indicates the decussating fibres of von Wilbrand's knee that detour into the fellow optic nerve.

ectodermal origin as the neurones and glial cells. During the 8th and 9th months mesodermal microglia appear and mesodermal elements also consolidate the structure of the lamina cribrosa. During this time the optic nerve increases in both diameter and length so that at birth it is approximately 2 mm in diameter and 24 mm long.

After the complete visual pathway has developed, myelination of nerve fibres occurs in the reverse direction to their growth. Myelination is wholly dependent on oligodendrocytes, and is first evident in the lateral geniculate bodies at about the 5th month. By the 6th month myelin reaches the optic tracts and chiasm and is apparent in the optic nerve by the 8th month. It slowly reaches the lamina cribrosa at or shortly after birth at which point the process normally ceases. In the phase of early postnatal visual development further myelination of the intra-orbital optic nerve occurs in tandem with myelination of the posterior pathways.

Melanin is thought to play a role in axonal guidance during development of the anterior visual pathways and major abnor-

11

malities of projection arise in human albinos (both oculocutaneous and ocular forms). The majority of fibres originating in the temporal retina are misdirected and decussate to the opposite lateral geniculate nucleus along with those from the nasal retina.[8] As a result, each hemisphere receives predominantly monocular input from the contralateral eye and failure to develop normal binocular function may explain in part the high frequency of strabismus and amblyopia in these patients.

Disruption of the process of controlled axonal loss in the second trimester of pregnancy explains the dysplastic syndromes involving one or both optic nerves, the chiasm, and other forebrain structures including the septum pellucidum and hypothalamus. For example, optic nerve hypoplasia may arise as a result of excess loss of axons during this period, although how this relates to specific teratogenic insults such as maternal alcohol and drug abuse is not clear. When the chiasm itself is dysplastic, there will be no decussation at all with retinofugal fibres projecting exclusively to the ipsilateral hemisphere. Such patients may not only have a bitemporal hemianopia but frequently have congenital see-saw nystagmus.[9] The congenital nystagmus in these patients may reflect abnormalities in extrageniculo-striate projections to subcortical structures. Because the nasal and temporal hemifields split the retina across the fovea and not across the optic nerve head, a very specific abnormality of the optic nerve head is seen when there is an absence or loss of crossing fibres. The optic nerve head will have deficient neuroretinal tissue at both nasal and temporal sides where nerve fibres serving the temporal hemifield enter, but not superiorly or inferiorly where fibres from the nasal hemifield enter. This is known as a "bow-tie" disc or hemioptic hypoplasia when the cause is developmental. The appearance may be seen in some congenital retrogeniculate lesions, reflecting the possibility of intrauterine trans-synaptic degeneration.[10]

1.4   The posterior visual pathways: optic tract, lateral geniculate nucleus, visual radiations, and visual cortex

Optic tracts

The optic tracts form immediately posterior to the chiasm as retinofugal fibres pass posteriorly around the cerebral peduncles.

The third ventricle lies superiorly, and the pituitary stalk medially. The uncal gyrus of the temporal lobe lies laterally. Ninety per cent of the fibres terminate in the ipsilateral lateral geniculate nucleus of the thalamus. The remainder are divided between those serving the afferent limb of the pupillomotor reflex which leave the tract to terminate in the pretectal nuclei of the rostral midbrain and others which synapse in the superior colliculus, the hypothalamus, and the accessory optic system to serve foveational eye movements, neuroendocrine function (circadian rhythms), and optokinetic eye movements respectively.[11,12] These extrageniculate pathways are also of clinical importance in the residual vision of infants with major cortical abnormalities, and in the phenomena of "blindsight" and stato-kinetic visual dissociation.[13] Fibres from the superior retinas occupy the dorsomedial portion of the optic tract, while those from the inferior retinas occupy the ventrolateral tract.

Lateral geniculate nucleus

The lateral geniculate ganglion is a highly differentiated structure lying in the thalamus, the function of which is best considered as analogous to a relay station between retina and visual cortex. Crossed and uncrossed retinal fibres are organised into homonymous pairs. Six grey layers of cell bodies are discernible in humans. Crossing visual axons terminate in layers (also called laminae) 1, 4, and 6, while uncrossed ipsilateral axons end in layers 2, 3, and 5. Each layer contains a complete representation of the entire hemifield of vision. The receptive fields of the lateral geniculate nucleus (LGN) cells resemble very closely those of the retinal ganglion neurones (RGNs) which provide their input. Magnocellular RGNs project to layers 1 and 2; the smaller parvocellular neurones to layers 3, 4, 5 and 6. Central vision is thought to be mediated by the dorsal portion of the lateral geniculate ganglion whilst peripheral vision is mediated ventrally where the six laminae fuse to become four. All six laminae are folded about a central hilum resulting in an exceedingly complex three-dimensional retinotopic pattern. Fibres from the superior retina pass to the medial aspect whilst those from the inferior retina pass to the lateral, with the result that lesions of the lateral geniculate ganglion result in the most non-congruous hemianopias. It is intriguing to note that there are extensive projections of nerve fibres from the prestriate cortex back to the lateral geniculate

13

ganglion, but there is little evidence as yet of functions other than the transmission of visual information from eye to cortex.

The visual (optic) radiations

Myelinated fibres forming the geniculocalcarine tract exit from the dorsal aspect of the lateral geniculate ganglion to pass posteriorly and laterally to the ipsilateral occipital cortex. The most anterior and inferior fibres serving the upper visual quadrant form a loop reaching approximately 4 cm caudal to the anterior pole of the temporal lobe (Meyer's loop) by passing around the anterior tip of the temporal horn of the lateral ventricle whereas those serving the inferior quadrant pass on a more direct route through the parietal lobe. Typically, lesions of the anterior radiations give rise to sector shaped homonymous defects which spare the horizontal meridian – if the lower field is affected then parietal fibres have been damaged; when the upper field is abnormal, fibres within Meyer's loop in the temporal lobe have been affected.

Occipital cortex

The primary visual cortex (Brodmann area 17, or area V1) lies in the interhemispheric fissure in relation to the falx cerebri with a macular projection area extending laterally by about 1 cm on to the posterior cortical surface. Anteriorly, the primary visual cortex lies superior and inferior to the calcarine fissure to reach the splenium of the corpus callosum. The term "striate" cortex is also used: this denotes the fact that when viewed macroscopically, a section of the primary visual cortex shows a thin white band (stria of Gennari) of myelinated fibres within the cortical grey matter. At least 60% of the surface of the primary visual cortex is devoted to the representation of the central 10 degrees of vision, reflecting the superior acuity and colour vision capability of this part of the visual field.[14] In spite of the hemidecussation of the visual pathways at the chiasm, the visual fields in the cortex do not completely overlap. In the deepest, most anterior part of each hemisphere there is a region serving the temporal peripheral field in which the outermost 30 degrees are seen monocularly. This means that occasionally lesions of the anterior occipital cortex result in a monocular field defect in spite of the fact that the lesion is post-chiasmal, and that more posterior lesions may spare this temporal crescent to produce a non-congruous hemianopia.

At a histological level, the six fundamental layers of the primate neocortex contain further subdivisions in the primary visual cortex reflecting functional anatomy. Magnocellular cells of the lateral geniculate ganglion project to layer IVC alpha and those of the parvocellular stream project to layer IVC beta. Layer IVB includes the myelinated fibres referred to as the striae of Gennari. Axon terminals from the left and right eyes are not randomly distributed but are segregated into alternating parallel strips called ocular dominance columns which are only lacking at the monocular temporal crescent and at the cortical representation of the blind-spot. Cells in the primary visual cortex are further arranged into those which respond maximally to stationary stimuli of specific orientation (simple cells), those which respond maximally to movement (complex cells), and those which are selective for both orientation and dimension (hypercomplex or end-stopped cells). In addition, cortical cells fall into the discrete parvocellular and magnocellular subsets referred to above with the LGN P cells projecting to both blob cells and interblob cells within layer IVC beta – the former apparently serving colour-responsive functions. Binocular integration occurs for the first time in the visual system in cells receiving inputs from monocular cells in layer IV.[15]

Visual association areas

Further analysis, recognition, and interpretation of afferent visual information takes place in the extrastriate (prestriate) cortex. These higher visual association areas are referred to as Brodmann areas 18 and 19. Current understanding of the anatomy and physiology of these areas depends almost entirely on animal models of great complexity, where the terms areas V2, V3, V4, and V5 (or MT standing for middle temporal) are used. Areas 17, 18, and 19 in one hemisphere are extensively interconnected with equivalent areas in the other hemisphere, principally via the splenium of the corpus callosum. Because the human cortex is a great deal larger and more complex than that of any animal model, the anatomical location of the human homologues of these areas remains to be elucidated fully. At a very simplistic level it is helpful to imagine that cortical area V1 projects via area V2 to two principal extrastriate territories: V4, served by the parvocellular system, and concerned

15

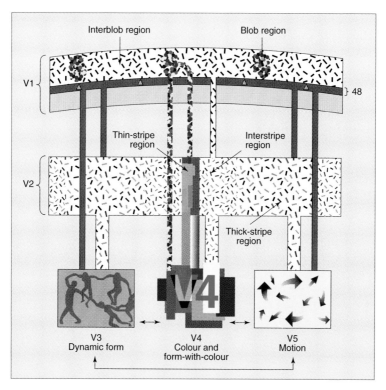

Figure 1.7   Visual perception at the cortical level. Mitochondrial cytochrome oxidase is present in high concentrations in highly metabolically active cells, and this enzyme has been used to label "hot" cells in the visual cortex. This has shown that cells in the visual cortex can be pigeon-holed into "blob" and "interblob" regions; blob cells exist as large columns, particularly in layers 2 and 3 of the visual cortex, and receive information from the parvocellular neurones in the LGN. Magnocellular structures synapse in layer 4B of V1 and connect with areas V5 and V3.

with colour and form (the "what?" area), and V5 (MT), served by the magnocellular system, and concerned with motion (the "where?" area).[16,17]

Vascular supply of the post-chiasmal pathways

The optic tract and lateral geniculate ganglion receive a dual blood supply from the anterior choroidal artery which is a direct branch of the internal carotid, and deep perforating thalamogeniculate branches of the posterior cerebral. The optic radiations also receive a supply from both the posterior cerebral

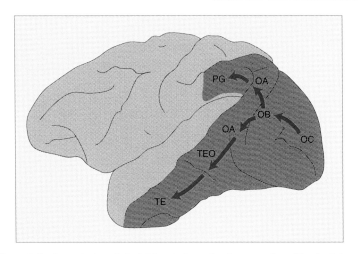

Figure 1.8 Lateral view of the left hemisphere of a rhesus monkey. The shaded area defines cortical visual tissue in the occipital, temporal, and parietal lobes. Arrows schematise two cortical visual pathways, each beginning in the primary visual cortex (area OC), diverging within the prestriate cortex (areas OB and OA), and then coursing either ventrally into the inferior temporal cortex (areas TEO and TE) or dorsally into the inferior parietal cortex (area PG). Both cortical visual pathways are crucial for higher visual function, the ventral pathway for object vision and the dorsal pathway for spatial vision.

artery inferiorly and the middle cerebral superiorly. The occipital cortex principally derives its supply from parieto-occipital (superiorly), calcarine (centrally), and posterior temporal (inferiorly) branches of the posterior cerebral. However, at the occipital pole there is a rich anastomotic network incorporating terminal branches of the middle cerebral artery. This configuration may explain the preservation of macular vision which is sometimes found in hemianopic field defects arising from vascular occlusion of posterior cerebral circulation to the occipital cortex – so-called "macular sparing".[19]

Acknowledgements

Figure 1.1 is reproduced from Acheson JF and Sanders MD. *Common problems in neuro-ophthalmology*. London: WB Saunders, 1997. Figure 1.2 is reproduced from Lee WR. *Ophthalmic histopathology*. Berlin: Springer-Verlag, 1993. Figure 1.3 is reproduced from Olver JM, Spalton DJ, McCartney AC. Quantitative

17

morphology of human retrolaminar optic nerve vasculature. *Invest Ophthalmol Vis Sci* 1994;**35**(11):3858–66. Figure 1.4 is after Glaser JS. *Neuro-ophthalmology,* 2nd edn. Philadelphia: Lippincott, 1990. Figure 1.5 is reproduced from Gross CG. *Brain, vision and memory – tales in the history of neuroscience.* Boston, MA: MIT Press, 1998: 66. Figure 1.6 is reproduced from Polyak S. *The vertebrate visual system.* Chicago: Chicago University Press, 1957. Figure 1.7 is reproduced from Zeki S. *A vision of the brain.* Oxford: Blackwell, 1993. Figure 1.8 is after Mishkin M, Ungerlieder LG, Macko K. Object vision and spatial vision: two cortical pathways. *Trends Neurosci* 1983;**6**:414–17.

1 Sadun AA. Parallel processing in the human visual system: a new perspective. *Neuro-Ophthalmol* 1986;**6**:351–2.

2 Merigan WH, Maunsell JHR. How parallel are the primate visual pathways? *Ann Rev Neuro Sci* 1993;**16**:369–402.

3 Maunsell JHR. Functional visual streams. *Curr Opin Neurobiol* 1992; **2**:506–10.

4 Ogden TE. Nerve fibre layer of the primate retina: morphometric analysis. *Invest Ophthalmol Vis Sci* 1984;**25**:19–29.

5 Plant GT, Perry VH. The anatomical basis of the caecocentral scotoma – new observations and a review. *Brain* 1990;**113**:1441–57.

6 Olver JM, Spalton DJ, McCartney AC. Quantitative morphology of human retrolaminar optic nerve vasculature. *Invest Ophthalmol Vis Sci* 1994;**35**(11):3858–66.

7 Hoyt CS, Good WV. Do we really understand the difference between optic nerve hypoplasia and atrophy? *Eye* 1992;**6**(2):201–4.

8 Apkarian P, Shallo-Hoffman J. VEP projections in congenital nystagmus; VEP asymmetry in albinism: a comparison study [published erratum appears in *Invest Ophthalmol Vis Sci* 1992;**33**(3): 691–2] *Invest Ophthalmol Vis Sci* 1991;**32**(9):2653–61.

9 Apkarian P, Bour LJ, Barth PG, Wenniger-Prick L, Verbeeten B Jr. Non-decussating retinal-fugal fibre syndrome. An inborn achiasmatic malformation associated with visuotopic misrouting, visual evoked potential ipsilateral asymmetry and nystagmus. *Brain* 1995;**118**(5): 1195–216.

10 Novakovic P, Taylor DS, Hoyt WF. Localising patterns of optic nerve hypoplasia – retina to occipital lobe. *Br J Ophthalmol* 1988;**72**(3): 176–82.

11 Sadun AA, Johnson BM, Smith LEH. Neuroanatomy of the human visual system. Part II: Retinal projections to the superior colliculus and pulvinar. *Neuro-Ophthalmol* 1986;**6**:363–70.

12 Sadun AA, Johnson BM, Schaechter JD. Neuroanatomy of the human visual system. Part III: Three retinal projections to the hypothalamus. *Neuro-Ophthalmol* 1986;**6**:371–9.

13 Zeki S, Ffytche DH. The Riddoch syndrome: insights into the neurobiology of conscious vision. *Brain* 1998;**121**:25–45.
14 Horton JC, Hoyt WF. The representation of the visual field in the human striate cortex: a revision of the classic Holmes map. *Arch Ophthalmol* 1991;**109**:816–24.
15 Horton JC. The central visual pathways. In: Hart WM. *Adler's Physiology of the Eye*, 9th edn. St Louis: Mosby Year Book, 1992: 728–72.
16 Livingstone M, Hubel D. Segregation of form, color, movement, and depth: Anatomy, physiology, and perception. *Science* 1988;**240**:740–9.
17 Zeki S, Watson JD, Lueck CJ, Friston KJ, Kennard C, Frakowiak RS. A direct demonstration of functional specialization in human visual cortex. *J Neurosci* 1991;**11**:641–9.
18 Mishkin M, Ungerlieder LG, Macko K. Object vision and spatial vision: two cortical pathways. *Trends Neurosci* 1983;**6**:414–17.
19 Smith CG, Richardson WFG. The course and distribution of the arteries supplying the visual (striate) cortex. *Am J Ophthalmol* 1966; **67**:139.

2: Clinical examination and investigation techniques

JF ACHESON

2.1 The visual sensory system
2.2 Specialised investigations in neuro-ophthalmology

2.1 The visual sensory system

Visual acuity testing

Although acuity testing only measures the central 1–2 degrees of field at 100% contrast, this measurement of visual health is almost universally understood and changing levels of performance measured in this way sometimes assume great medicolegal significance. None the less, it is always important to remember that there are many limitations to the accuracy and reproducibility of acuity levels achieved on a Snellen chart, and in vision science LogMAR charts are always preferred.[1,2]

Some patients experience difficulty in reading out of proportion to their optically corrected 6 metre Snellen acuity as a result of parafoveal scotomata or poor gaze holding in certain eye movement disorders.

Factors influencing visual acuity

In order to achieve peak performance referred to as normal visual acuity, all optical, anatomical, and physiological elements must themselves perform normally.[3] For example, acuity is readily degraded by refractive error so that 1 dioptre of defocus will reduce the Snellen fraction to about 0.3. Young hypermetropes (hyperopes)

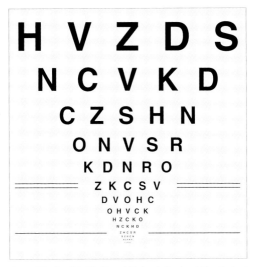

Figure 2.1   The LogMAR (Log Minimal Angle of Resolution) chart.

can accommodate to overcome their own refractive error, but myopes and presbyopes cannot. A pin-hole is very helpful but it is important to remember its limitations: only 4 dioptres of spherical and cylindrical error may be corrected, so an up-to-date refraction is essential in all cases of unexplained visual loss.

Photostress testing, Amsler grid, and acuity testing at reduced illumination

In all instances of deficient vision the clinician must ask whether the observed pathology matches the degree of visual loss. Normally this question can be easily answered by examining the eye, but it is not unusual for a patient to have an apparently normal eye and yet still have poor vision. When this occurs in one eye only the problem probably will be localised to the optic nerve, especially when there is a marked colour vision deficit and a relative afferent pupil defect. However, subtle retinal pathology involving the fovea and central vision may easily be overlooked and simple tests to distinguish macular from optic nerve lesions are sometimes helpful before recourse to more sophisticated electrodiagnostic methods.

In the photostress test the subject fixates on a bright light for a defined period of time (about 30 seconds) and the time to recovery of acuity to the pretest level after eventual disappearance of the induced positive scotoma is measured. In lesions of the choroid,

21

retinal pigment epithelium or retinal photoreceptors, recovery from this bleaching is greatly prolonged, whereas in optic nerve disease photostressing does not produce the same effect as function is not dependent on the rapid functioning of the visual cycle.

The Amsler grid is a coarse high contrast grid against which the small paracentral scotomas of macular disease can readily be seen.

A special clinical difficulty commonly arises in the discrimination between poor uniocular vision due to amblyopia ("lazy eye") of any cause which the adult patient may only later become aware of, and an acquired cause of visual loss without evident intraocular pathology. When illumination is reduced (for example by using a standard neutral density filter), acuity is preserved in eyes with longstanding visual loss due to amblyopia, but is markedly degraded in an acquired optic neuropathy: this test is sometimes invaluable in distinguishing amblyopia from, for example, optic neuritis. One other feature of the amblyopic eye is that on single letter Snellen chart testing, acuity improves on the single letter per line format: this phenomenon is known as crowding.

Further psychophysical tests of vision

Contrast sensitivity

The patient who complains of "faded" vision but who has a normal (high contrast) Snellen acuity can readily be shown to have defects in contrast sensitivity. The level of contrast at which a light and dark pattern is first discriminated is the contrast threshold. No consistent discrimination occurs for contrast below the subject's threshold for a particular spatial frequency. High spatial frequencies and very low spatial frequencies require higher contrast for resolution. Contrast sensitivity is measured as the reciprocal of contrast threshold using sine wave (sinusoidal) gratings showing gradual change from light to dark. Measurement aims to record the contrast threshold over a range of spatial frequencies using gratings of different contrast levels. Pathological reduction in contrast sensitivity occurs in developmental and acquired visual defects when the contrast threshold can be raised for low, high or all spatial frequencies depending on the underlying cause.[4]

User-friendly book-mounted charts introduced by Arden and Regan are commercially available. Wall-mounted charts are also useful; for example the VisTech and Pelli–Robson systems. In a

VisTech chart photographs of sinusoidal gratings are presented and thresholds for different spatial frequencies are determined by the subject recognising the correct orientation of the stripes, while in the simpler Pelli–Robson chart standard sized optotypes of uniform spatial frequency are presented with decreasing contrast as the subject reads along a line allowing threshold detection.

In visual science contrast sensitivity forms the basis of one of the most important psychophysical methods for measuring visual function: for example, allowing the demonstration that neurones of the visual system are sensitive to limited ranges of spatial frequency and orientation. In clinical practice these methods allow the detection of otherwise subclinical pathology and offer a sensitive way of following patients with chronic disease.

Colour vision

It is a characteristic of certain disorders of the anterior visual pathways that sensitivity to hue discrimination (colour vision) may be impaired while luminance and contrast based functions (acuity) are preserved.[5]

The inherited dyschromatopsias are binocular, symmetrical, and do not change over time. Monochromats have major cone defects and have poor acuity as well, but dichromats and anomalous trichromats have normal acuity.

Acquired dyschromatopsias are different from congenital defects in several respects. First, they are noticeable to the subject. Secondly, they may be monocular or even restricted to one part of the visual field. Thirdly, although colour defects may be much more marked than acuity defects, acuity is generally reduced to some degree. According to Kollner's rule, patients with neural disorders have a preponderance of damage to red–green discrimination with preservation of blue–yellow discrimination (type I and II defects), while those with retinal and choroidal disease may show selective loss of blue–yellow discrimination (type III defects).

However, some optic neuropathies – especially those associated with preserved acuity – may show type III defects. Because blue cones are not found in the central 0.5 degrees of field, disease processes which selectively damage the extrafoveal visual field will leave the patient with normal acuity and abnormal blue–yellow discrimination. Examples of this include glaucoma, dominant optic atrophy, chronic papilloedema, and early chloroquine retinal toxicity. More typically, optic neuropathies which involve the fibres of the foveal projection, such as retrobulbar neuritis, Leber's disease, and extrinsic compression, will damage neural elements serving foveal function, and green–red discrimination will be damaged, often out of proportion to acuity loss.

Formal colour vision testing using spectral light sources graded for luminance changes is very demanding and time consuming, and not very practicable in the clinical setting. Pseudo-isochromatic plates are very widely used because of their portability, low cost, and ease of use. The plates consist of a series of dots of various colours and sizes that are clustered together into carefully arranged patterns consisting of various hues. These hues can readily be distinguished by a normal trichromat but not by those with defective colour vision. The patterns form highly legible figures which are visible even to those with relatively poor acuity. An initial test plate excludes subjects whose acuity or reading skills do not allow them to perform the test. Commercially available pseudo-isochromatic plates (Ishihara and Hardy, Ritter, Read (HRR) plates) are designed to detect individuals with congenital dyschromatopsias, but do not allow protan–deutan distinctions or the separation of anomalous trichromats from dichromats. They are also of practical use in the qualitative assessment of acquired colour defects. A greater quantitative element is supplied by the Farnsworth–Munsell 100-hue test in which the subject is required to arrange a series of coloured discs in sequence between pairs of reference discs. The order of discs is then plotted in a circular diagram so that the degree of error is represented by points far away from the centre of the diagram. Characteristic patterns for errors along the red–green and blue–yellow axis will emerge allowing full characterisation of the dyschromatopsia. Even with automated, computer assisted versions however, this test is inconvenient and time consuming, and is not greatly used for this reason. The Farnsworth D-15 (dichotomous) panel test simplifies matters by recording confusions in the allocation of non-adjacent hues into their correct colour grouping.

Visual field testing

The analysis of the visual fields retains central importance in the localisation of defects in the visual system, and for monitoring the natural history of a condition and responses to therapy. Simple confrontation testing (qualitative) remains useful in clinic-based and bedside topical diagnosis, but semi-quantitative and quantitative methods are essential for accurate documentation, detection of more subtle defects, and for assessing progress. The diagnostic value of field testing rests on the principle of the retino-topic organisation of the afferent visual system whereby nerve fibres from retinal ganglion cells serving defined parts of the visual field project in an anatomically consistent arrangement (see Chapter 1).

In testing the visual field it is helpful to employ Traquair's analogy of the hill of vision. The field is represented as a three-dimensional hill with the base plane representing the horizontal and vertical dimensions of visual space and the hill representing the sensitivity of the retina to stimulation by a focal light at different places. At the pinnacle of the hill is the fovea where even the dimmest and smallest target can be detected. This concept allows for the representation of relative field loss as alteration in the slope of the hill, as well as constriction ("coast erosion"), and absolute loss (the blindspot for example). Lines joining points of equal sensitivity are isopters, and using the standard manual perimeter (Goldmann), the isopters are determined either by moving a spot of light from periphery to centre until it hits the hill and is perceived (kinetic testing), or by increasing the intensity of stimulus at one spot until threshold is reached (static testing). The concept of the hill of vision is also useful in confrontation testing, where relative defects can be detected by eliciting differential brightness of say a hand, or a red bottle top in opposite hemifields. In other individuals, however, it is not practicable to depend on the subject's conscious response, and an involuntary saccadic eye movement to fixate on a peripherally placed stimulus may serve as a sensitive test for obtunded or preverbal patients.

Quantitative perimetry is made difficult by the need for highly trained and experienced perimetrists who can reliably distinguish between pathology and artifact, and automated perimetry machines are now widely available. Ease of data storage and standardisation of presentation are advantages. With increasing sensitivity, however, specificity is lost and it is important to use a test technique that supports practical management decisions. Many automated systems are primarily designed for the detection of subclinical disease states which will not be detectable by confrontation, in particular early glaucomatous optic neuropathy, and are not necessarily suitable for characterising patterns of field defect which is so important in topical neuro-ophthalmic diagnosis. Other

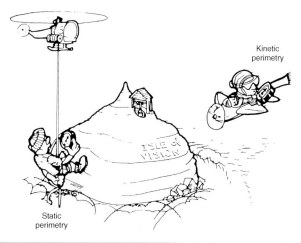

Kinetic
perimetry

Static
perimetry

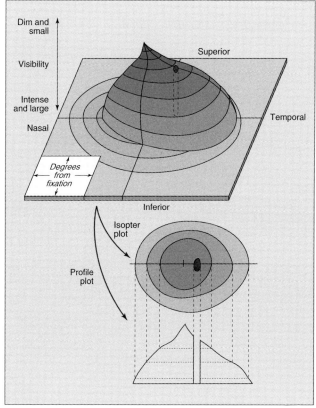

26

Some limitations of automated perimetry in neuro-ophthalmology

- Systemic disease increases patient fatigue and short term fluctuation effects
- Fixation testing strategies are inappropriate in presence of dense temporal defects
- Stato-kinetic dissociation may mask significant defects

Table 2.1   Specific types of field loss in optic nerve disease

Field defect	Pathophysiology	Common causes
Arcuate scotoma	Retinal nerve fibre bundle damage selectively involving fibres entering disc at 12 o'clock and 6 o'clock	Glaucoma, optic disc drusen, optic neuritis, ischaemic lesions
Centrocaecal scotoma	Selective damage to fibres of foveal and centrocaecal projections serving central vision and lying in the temporal side of the anterior optic nerve	Leber's hereditary optic neuropathy, toxic optic neuropathies – ethambutol, ethanol, methanol, tobacco, rarely optic neuritis
Altitudinal scotoma	Selective damage to upper or lower poles of the optic nerve: reflecting susceptibility at these points to reduced vascular perfusion pressure in the anastomotic circle of Zinn–Haller deriving from branches of the short posterior ciliary vessels and lying at the level of the lamina cribrosa	Anterior ischaemic optic neuropathy, rarely optic neuritis and compressive lesions

problems include patient learning effects, physiological variation in field performance over time, fatigue, and stato-kinetic dissociation.[6,7] In addition, test strategies emphasise threshold changes across the horizontal meridian, but in neuro-ophthalmic assessment, the vertical meridian is of crucial diagnostic

Figure 2.2   The "island" or "hill" of vision proposed by Traquair is surrounded by a "sea of blindness". The height of the island represents increasing sensitivity. Using kinetic perimetry, the island is intercepted by a moving target of fixed size. Using static perimetry, a target's visibility is increased in size or luminosity until it descends on to the island. The blindspot located 15 degrees temporal to fixation is absolute, creating a small "well" in the sensitivity contour.

Table 2.2 Confrontation techniques in visual field testing

Confrontation with neurological pin-heads
Visually elicited eye movements
   Infants
   Obtunded adults
Finger mimicking
   Preverbal children
   Dysphasic adults
Hand and colour comparison
   Children and adults
Blinking to menace and flashing lights
   Children and obtunded adults

importance, and fixation testing strategies rely on repeated blindspot checking which is, of course, lost in bitemporal defects of chiasmal disease.

2.2   Specialised investigations in neuro-ophthalmology

Fluorescein angiography

Fluorescein angiography provides an important adjunct to the ophthalmoscopy of diseases of the retina and the optic nerve head by demonstrating evidence of disease activity and by providing a permanent record. In the evaluation of optic disc swelling, true disc oedema can be distinguished from the pseudopapilloedema of buried optic disc drusen or elevated discs in hypermetropic eyes by demonstrating the presence of dilated capillaries on the disc surface during the arterial phase of the angiogram, and hyperfluorescence in the late venous phase. In addition, buried disc drusen may fluoresce without any injection of dye – a phenomenon known as autofluorescence – thus avoiding unnecessary imaging and cerebrospinal fluid (CSF) studies, and sometimes shunting procedures as well. Further examples are given in Table 2.3.

Clinical electrophysiology

Psychophysical methods of acuity measurement, contrast function, motion detection, perimetry and colour vision all depend on a stimulus–response paradigm which is mediated by the subject's conscious understanding of the test, and certain assumptions must be made about the correlation of these stimulus–reponse properties

Table 2.3   Selected indications for fluorescein angiography in neuro-ophthalmology

Clinical problem	Comment
Optic disc swelling	Distinction between true acquired pathological disc swelling of raised intracranial pressure or local disease and pseudopapilloedema of hypermetropic eyes, buried disc drusen, and other anomalies
Multifocal cerebral white matter lesions or unexplained optic neuropathy	Subtle or subclinical retinal vasculitis indicates an inflammatory cause (multiple sclerosis, sarcoidosis or Behçet's)
Unexplained visual acuity loss with a central scotoma	Subtle macular pathology (age-related macular degeneration, branch retinal vein occlusion, retinal dystrophies)
Neuromuscular disease	Mild or severe forms of retinal pigment epithelial degeneration well shown in the mitochondrial myopathies (Kearnes–Sayre syndrome).
Unexplained cranial nerve palsies	Demonstration of choroidal abnormalities in the uveo-meningeal syndromes (Vogt–Koyanagi–Harada syndrome, Behçet's, sarcoidosis, non–Hodgkin's lymphoma, metastatic carcinoma)

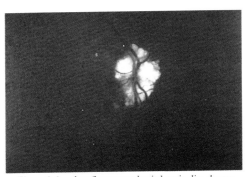

Figure 2.3   Autofluorescent buried optic disc drusen.

to physiological events. The clinical electrophysiology of vision bypasses this area of theoretical and practical complexity and allows closer correlation with physiological functions. There is the added advantage of being suitable for the assessment of vision in preverbal children, and in neurologically impaired subjects. The chief disadvantage is the high degree of technical expertise required to give consistent results, and for this reason tests are used selectively.

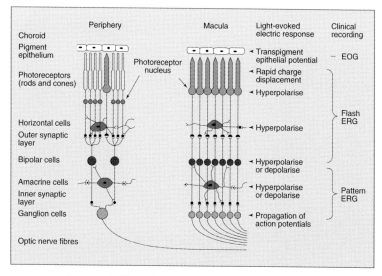

Figure 2.4   Electrophysiological recording of visual function.

Visual evoked potentials

Following repetitive visual stimulation using flashes of light or sudden changes in a grid pattern, a cortical potential is detectable which may be summated and averaged using microprocessors after repeated testing to yield the visual evoked cortical potential (VECP) or visual evoked response (VER). The VER reflects the integrity of the central visual field throughout the entire afferent visual system but is non-specific in localising a lesion to the retina, optic nerve or cortex. The VER primarily represents the central visual field for the reason that most of the occipital cortex is concerned with the central 10 degrees, and also that the most central field has the most posterior location in the cortex and is therefore the most detectable. A flash generated VER is stimulated by luminance change while a pattern VER is stimulated by contrast change. The complex waveform is described in terms of amplitude and latency according to characteristics of the P_1 wave which is a large positive deflection occurring at around 100 msec. Amplitude varies widely amongst normal subjects but latency is constant.

Pathological conditions of the anterior visual pathways yield relatively non-specific abnormalities of the VER, but the test is none the less useful, especially when carried out in conjunction with flash and pattern generated electroretinograms (see below).

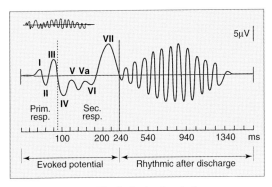

Figure 2.5   The flash visual evoked response.

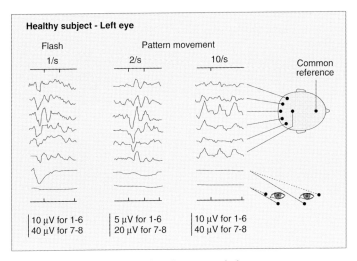

Figure 2.6   Flash and pattern evoked responses.

Latency delay with relative amplitude preservation is found in demyelination, even long after the acute episode and following visual recovery and also in optic nerve compression. Amplitude reduction is a feature of ischaemic optic neuropathy and other conditions where axonal loss is prominent compared to conduction block. By careful choice of stimulus parameters (check size and reversal speed in the pattern-generated VEP), the effects of optical blurring can be minimised and the test made sufficiently sensitive to be useful in those patients with moderate or minimal acuity loss.

31

Additional specificity can be achieved by half-field testing whereby differences in amplitude and latency recorded from each hemisphere after uniocular stimulation can be used to assess abnormalities of the optic chiasm. Further refinements in VER techniques, which are currently undergoing clinical evaluation, include differential testing of the parvo- and magnocellular systems by use of test targets which selectively stimulate chromatic, temporal, and spatial functions, and also the discrimination between striate, extrastriate, and subcortical responses.

Electroretinography

Stimulation of the eye with either a flash or a pattern reversal system results in a recordable potential from the retina which has two principle components: the a-wave which reflects the activity of the photoreceptors, and the b-wave which arises from the inner nuclear layer and the Müller cells.

Disorders predominantly involving cones can be distinguished from those involving rods by performing the test in light (photopic) and dark (scotopic) conditions. In primary retinal diseases, such as diabetic retinopathy, pigmentary retinopathies and dystrophies, and in toxic degenerations, both the a-wave and the b-wave are abnormal.[8] Exceptions to this are seen in central retinal artery occlusion where in the acute phase the photoreceptors which derive their blood supply from the choriocapillaris are preserved and therefore the a-wave persists while the b-wave is extinguished. Superimposed on the b-wave in a normal retina are a series of rhythmic oscillations referred to as oscillatory potentials which may be of diagnostic importance when lost in the early stages of both diabetic retinopathy and in pigmentary retinopathies. When visual loss results from diseases which involve the ganglion cells or optic nerve, such as Tay–Sachs disease, glaucoma or optic neuritis, the ERG in response to flashes of light is usually normal. Only in advanced cases of retinal ganglion cell loss does the flash ERG become abnormal, as a result of secondary trans-synaptic degeneration of outer retinal elements (bipolar cells and photoreceptors).

In practice, the clinician must distinguish between visual acuity loss of retinal and optic nerve origin.[9] Sometimes, a pattern ERG (PERG) is useful. Just as the use of pattern reversal stimuli instead of flash offers greater sensitivity in the VEP, so it does with the ERG. Although the origins of the PERG are not entirely clear, it is accepted that the response does arise from retinal structures proximal to the photoreceptors, and it is this anatomical localisation which, together with the fact that pattern reversal stimuli test the central retina only, gives the test its potential power. Unlike the flash ERG, the late components of the PERG are abnormal in optic nerve and retinal ganglion cell layer disorders. Therefore, the PERG may be of value in discriminating subtle cases of central visual loss of central retinal origin, when early and late components will be abnormal from visual loss of optic nerve origin when the late component alone is abnormal. Unfortunately, the technical difficulties associated with obtaining reproducible PERG results are considerable, and this useful investigation is not as yet widely available. By using specialised light projection systems it is possible to test cone function by projecting a spot stimulus to the fovea rather than across the entire field (ganzfield) and foveal ERGs may develop as an alternative to the PERG. With the increasing recognition that subclinical abnormalities of retinal function may be of diagnostic importance in, for example, the tapeto-retinal degenerations and in the mitochondrial cytopathies, the use of electroretinography is likely to gain in importance in clinical neuro-ophthalmology.[10,11]

Electro-oculography

The human eye behaves like a dipole with a difference in electrical potential between the cornea and the retina of about 6 mV. Movements of the eye cause changes of the potential in one electrode placed near the inner canthus relative to another one placed near the outer canthus. This record of eye movement is called the electro-oculogram, or EOG. The EOG consists of two separate potentials, one that is insensitive and another that is sensitive to light. Under usual recording conditions the potential is measured in the dark adapted eye and then again 10–15 minutes after exposure to light (the EOG light rise). The ratio of peak voltage obtained in the light rise potential over the minimum voltage obtained in the dark trough is usually greater than 1.8.

The dark adapted EOG derives from the retinal pigment epithelium and the light rise from a combination of rods and cones. Typically the ERG is abnormal in conditions when the EOG is abnormal with important exceptions which include Best's disease (including carriers) and fundus flavimaculatus.

33

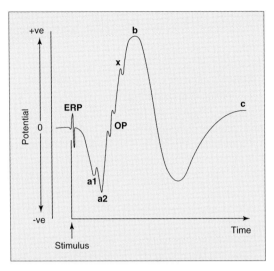

Figure 2.7 The flash electroretinograph. (ERP=Early Receptor Potential; OP= Oscillatory Potentials)

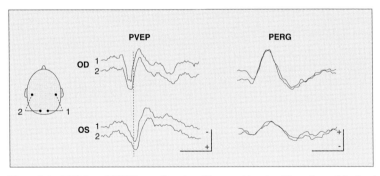

Figure 2.8 PERG and PVEP recordings in a 39-year-old male with moderate left visual impairment (acuity reduced to 6/12). The left eye PVEP shows a 20 ms delay but the PERG shows a moderate P50 component abnormality in keeping with dysfunction distal to the optic nerve: the diagnosis was central serous retinopathy.

Ultrasound, Doppler and colour Doppler flow mapping (colour Doppler imaging)

Real-time B-mode ultrasound is an important alternative to CT scanning in the examination of orbital structures, and in particular the anterior optic nerve, where buried drusen causing pseudopapilloedema, and optic nerve sheath distension in chronic papilloedema can readily be demonstrated.[12] Disc swelling due to

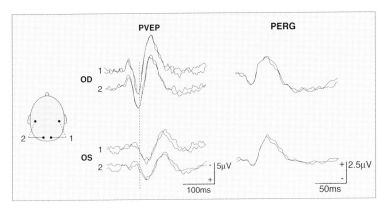

Figure 2.9   PERG and PVEP recordings in a 35-year-old male with asymptomatic optic disc pallor (normal acuities). Left eye PVEP markedly delayed; left eye PERG shows reduced N95 component consistent with retinal ganglion cell or nerve fibre loss.

local scleral or optic nerve sheath swelling can also be shown (scleritis and perineuritis), and also optic nerve calcification in cases where the distinction between meningioma and glioma is difficult.

However, it is in investigation of patients with vascular disease that sonographic methods have the most to offer. Although selective intra-arterial angiography may remain the definitive examination technique for extracranial carotid disease, sonographic techniques have reached the point where non-invasive assessment is sufficiently accurate to be useful in screening for atherosclerotic disease, allowing the use of angiography, either by intravenous digital subtraction or by arterial cannulation, to be restricted to selected cases. Indirect tests of vascular patency such as simple Doppler imaging of directional blood flow have been superseded by direct B-mode ultrasonographic scanning of the vascular lumen and atherosclerotic plaque. The Duplex scanner combines simultaneous real-time B-mode arterial images and pulsed Doppler so that both lumen patency and flow velocity can be estimated. Interpretative caution is required, however, as these methods do not allow the distinction to be made between a severe stenosis and complete occlusion, and there may be difficulties in distinguishing between internal and external carotid lesions in patients with a high bifurcation, and in obtaining adequate studies in the obese patient.[13] Other non-invasive tests of extracranial carotid function may also be useful, ranging from simple observation of central

35

retinal artery patency as the intraocular pressure is raised in ophthalmodynanometry, to ocular suction cup devices in ophthalmo-pneumoplethysmography.

Colour Doppler flow mapping is a further refinement where the spatial and temporal distribution of the colour-coded Doppler signal can be visualised in real time and superimposed on a high resolution grey scale image of the tissue and vessel morphology. This has been applied to the study of extracranial carotid disease, but may be of greater clinical value in the assessment of vascular lesions of the cavernous sinus and orbit. The demonstration of reversed blood flow with an arterial waveform in the superior ophthalmic vein is of diagnostic importance in patients with carotid–cavernous and dural fistulas, and is a parameter which can be used to monitor clinical progress.[14] In addition, reduced ophthalmic artery blood flow may be shown in cases where chronic ocular ischaemia complicates occlusive carotid disease.[15] These developments have led investigators to study smaller and smaller vessels in the orbit, and in particular the central retinal artery and the short posterior ciliary arteries which supply the choroid and retrolaminar optic nerve.[16] However, reproducible results have been difficult to obtain as these vessels are multiple and there is considerable inter-individual variation in their disposition. In addition, the normal vascular lumen of a short posterior ciliary artery is too small to be measured by sonographic methods, so total blood flow measurements cannot reliably be obtained.

Neuro-imaging

The use of imaging in the assessment of visual failure requires an appreciation of the complementary roles of MR and CT, and in particular, an understanding of the contribution specific MR imaging strategies and sequences can make to the solution of specific clinical problems.[17] In general terms, MR is preferable to CT with some important exceptions, namely:

- Demonstration of bone lesions (fractures, neoplastic erosion).
- Acute haemorrhage (blood invisible on MR initially).
- MR contraindicated by cardiac pacemaker, transcutaneous neural stimulators, metallic intraocular foreign bodies, and magnetic aneurysm clips.

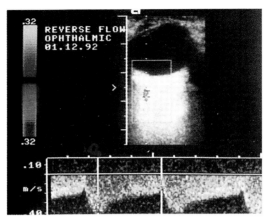

Figure 2.10   Orbital ultrasound study showing reversal (blue colour) within the ophthalmic artery in a patient with ipsilateral carotid artery occlusion.

- Definition of orbital structures (unless surface coils and fat suppression techniques available).
- Demonstration of dystrophic calcification in optic nerve head drusen and optic nerve sheath meningioma.

Intravenous injection of contrast enhancing agents (iodinated compounds for CT and paramagnetic gadolinium for MR) help the resolution of lesions associated with blood–brain barrier abnormalities or increased vasculature.

Some imaging considerations according to anatomical region

Globe MRI is contraindicated by the possibility of a ferro-magnetic foreign body, where torque created by the high magnetic field may dislodge the fragment and cause further intraocular damage. Titanium or cobalt-nickel retinal tacks, or intraocular lens loops made of platinum or titanium are not contraindications. CT is superior to MRI in retinoblastoma and astrocytic hamartoma because of the clinical importance of detecting intraocular calcification. MR may be useful in the assessment of solid retinal detachment as the paramagnetic properties of melanin in choroidal melanoma lead to bright signal T-1 weighted images. B-mode ultrasound remains the investigation of choice in most other posterior ocular segment diseases where there is media opacity.

37

Orbit Routine head CT scans do not give good orbital images, where special head positioning is required. Coronal imaging is preferable, but on CT this requires the patient to lie prone with the neck extended, which may not be well tolerated. With this method, the bony orbital walls, rectus muscles and their relationship to the optic nerves may all be studied. Computer facilitated three-dimensional image reconstruction is valuable in the assessment of facial and orbital trauma. CT will demonstrate the hyperostosis and calcification associated with a meningioma, and is suitable for the detection of both ferrous and non-ferrous foreign bodies with and without an acute haematoma.

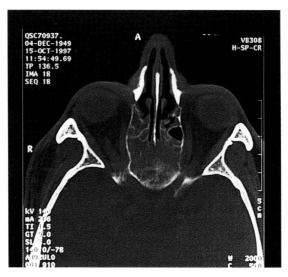

Figure 2.11   Axial CT scan of orbits (bone windows): extensive bone erosion associated with a malignant paranasal carcinoma in a patient presenting with a right compressive optic neuropathy.

Primary orbital tumours and metastases are also well seen on CT. However, in a number of specific instances, MR offers certain advantages, especially when high resolution is facilitated by the use of fat signal suppression techniques and headcoils. In cavernous haemangioma, the bright signal of T-2 and hypointense signal of T-1 sequences may allow radiographic distinction from a glioma or meningioma, which is valuable when the lesion is at a site inaccessible to biopsy, such as at the orbital apex. MR can identify feeder vessels in a lymphangioma prior to surgery and also distinguish fluid levels, septa, and lobulated structures, reflecting the non-encapsulated structure of this lesion. The superior ophthalmic vein is well seen on contrast enhanced CT and on MR: sudden worsening in a patient with carotid–cavernous fistula due to thrombosis of the superior ophthalmic vein may be indicated by a high signal on T-1 weighted images.

In primary optic nerve sheath meningiomas, gadolinium-enhanced MR is superior to CT in evaluating intracanalicular and intracranial extension, and also in distinguishing perioptic tumour growth from distal cystic change. Fat-suppression T-1 weighted imaging gives superior delineation of tumour surface adjacent to orbital fat, and demonstrates the tram-tracking sign characteristic of meningiomas by enhancing the contrast between tumour and the perineural subarachnoid space.[18] In optic glioma, MRI can distinguish between perineural growth giving rise to arachnoid gliomatosis and a dilated patulous optic nerve sheath.[19]

Inflammatory and neurodegenerative diseases of the optic nerve are also suitable for study with MR. Long areas of abnormal signal on fat-suppression short tau inversion (STIR) sequences in acute optic neuritis may correlate with poorer prognosis for visual recovery.[20] The absence of abnormal signals arising from the cerebrum and brain stem in Leber's hereditary optic neuropathy may help in the distinction from optic neuritis. Periventricular high signal lesions on T-2 weighted sequences are also seen in ischaemic gliosis, and therefore may lose clinical significance in subjects over the age of 40 years. Transient gadolinium leakage reflecting breakdown of the blood–brain barrier is seen in sarcoid optic neuropathy, and in the early stages of an episode of acute idiopathic optic neuritis. Gadolinium enhancement of a lesion which does not give rise to abnormal signal without the use of contrast is seen months after the onset of visual loss in radionecrosis of the anterior visual pathways.

Sellar and parasellar region   MRI is generally preferable to CT in the assessment of lesions in the sellar and parasellar regions for the following reasons: direct coronal images may be more readily obtained, interruption or invasion of the flow voids in the cavernous sinus and carotid artery by disease processes allow detailed imaging, CSF-neurovascular interfaces are clearly shown, subacute haemorrhage in pituitary apoplexy is easier to demonstrate, and finally meningeal enhancement distinct from bone signal is readily

Table 2.4 Some MRI features of optic nerve disease

A: Intrinsic lesions	
Optic neuritis	Increased signal on fat-suppression STIR sequences
Radionecrosis	Late gadolinium enhancement
Neurosarcoid	Meningeal enhancement associated with optic nerve signal
Optic glioma	Demonstration of perineural arachnoid gliomatosis
B: Extrinsic lesions	
Perioptic meningioma	Gadolinium enhancement and demonstration of intracranial extension in primary optic nerve sheath meningioma

seen. However, CT may supply additional information, for example detecting calcium in craniopharyngioma, hyperostosis in meningioma and bone distraction in nasopharyngeal carcinoma or metastases. Both MR and CT may fail to detect pituitary microadenomas or to allow the distinction from other intrasellar lesions such as pars intermedia cysts.

Posterior fossa MR offers advantages over CT in studying the brain stem and cerebellum because of the absence of beam hardening artifacts arising from the petrous ridge. However, MR artifacts may arise from pulsatile blood flow in the carotids, jugular, and torcula. Sagittal imaging from the mesencephalic junction to the foramen magnum is especially useful in patients with gaze palsies, internuclear ophthalmoplegia or nystagmus. Cryptic infratentorial arteriovenous malformations are well seen because of high signal arising from haemosiderin associated with previous overt or clinically silent haemorrhage. MR imaging may also show aberrant vessels at the pontomedullary junction in hemifacial spasm and in some cases of trigeminal neuralgia: such patients may benefit from decompression surgery. Magnetic resonance angiography and three-dimensional MR imaging are further refinements which are rapidly becoming available.

Further imaging techniques

Magnetic resonance angiography Selective intra-arterial angiography continues to set the gold standard for vascular imaging in the head and neck because of its excellent spatial resolution.

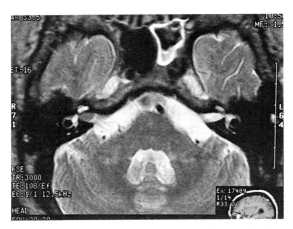

Figure 2.12   Posterior fossa axial MRI showing intracanalicular vestibular schwannoma in a patient with hemifacial spasm. This finding was probably coincidental: note the VIIth and VIIIth cranial nerves exiting the pons and passing across the pontine cistern (CSF is white in this sequence) to the internal acoustic meatus.

However, the infrequent but real risks of vascular damage, adverse systemic reactions, transient and permanent neurological defects, and even death have stimulated the development of alternative techniques. Intravenous contrast enhanced digital subtraction angiography (DSA) is limited by the need to insert central venous catheters, by poor image quality, and by systemic reactions. Ultrasonographic methods are non-invasive but are highly operator-dependent and limited in anatomical coverage because of the signal attenuating effects of bone.

Magnetic resonance angiography is a non-invasive technique whereby it is possible to generate high contrast between stationary tissue and flowing blood by suitable manipulation of imaging parameters. Interpretation depends on a computerised depiction of data based on the haemodynamic properties of flowing blood rather than on actual vessel anatomy. Because of the physiology of blood flow, the diameter of vessels may sometimes appear smaller on MRA techniques than with conventional arteriography, primarily because of the slower laminar flow near the vessel wall. As a result, aneurysms and ulceration of atheromatous plaques may not be well seen. There are extracranial applications for MRA as an adjunctive method for the study of carotid occlusive disease and dissections. Intracranial applications include the study of dural and carotid–cavernous fistula (although conventional angiography is

41

required to distinguish a direct carotid origin from one arising from a dural vessel, and to allow endovascular therapy), screening for intracranial aneurysms in high risk patients with positive family history, polycystic renal disease, fibromuscular dysplasia and aortic coarctation, and in the detection of supratentorial arteriovenous malformations, and perhaps most importantly, in the diagnosis of dural venous sinus obstruction by thrombus, infiltration or compression.[21]

Interventional neuroradiology The endovascular therapy of CNS vascular lesions has developed as the logical extension of refined diagnostic neuroangiography, employing advances in real-time imaging, new coaxial catheter systems, new embolic agents, and balloon techniques. The principle conditions in neuro-ophthalmology in which these methods are now important are direct carotid–cavernous fistula, dural arteriovenous fistulas involving the cavernous sinus, and intracranial aneurysms. In addition, patients with supratentorial and infratentorial arteriovenous malformations may present to the ophthalmologist, or require ophthalmic follow-up. The majority of these procedures on adults are performed with sedation only, using a transfemoral approach for catheterisation, and following anticoagulation with heparin. Transvenous approaches are reserved for patients with prior carotid ligation or other significant carotid pathology.

There is now abundant evidence that in carotid cavernous fistula of both traumatic and non-traumatic origin the prognosis for vision is much improved by treatment with these methods when compared to direct carotid ligation procedures. Simple reduction of the arterial pressure on its own will exacerbate ocular ischaemia, and it is only by closing a fistula directly that the venous pressure in eye and orbit can be reduced and normal perfusion gradients restored.[22] Indirect dural arteriovenous fistula results in a less severe initial clinical picture with insidious onset, but there may still be considerable ocular morbidity. Selective and superselective catheterisation of internal and external carotids bilaterally is required to assess the possibility of multiple feeder vessels and transarterial or transvenous embolisation routes employed. The treatment of intracranial aneuryms by interventional methods is reserved for those unsuitable for surgical clipping. This applies in particular to giant intracavernous and carotid–ophthalmic aneurysms. A detachable balloon is used either to embolise an

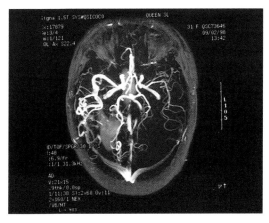

Figure 2.13   MR angiogram study showing axial view of circle of Willis with a large right posterior cerebral hemisphere arteriovenous malformation: note the dilated anomalous vessels peripherally – this patient had a homonymous hemianopia due to a spontaneous intracerebral haemorrhage.

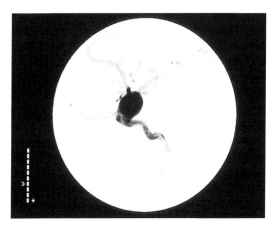

Figure 2.14   Intracavernous and suprasellar giant carotid aneurysm presenting with an optic neuropathy: note intraluminal material representing part of an endovascular embolisation procedure.

aneurysm or feeder vessels directly, or sometimes to occlude the internal carotid artery proximal to the neck of an aneurysm. Neuro-ophthalmic symptoms due to local cranial nerve compression resolve as the balloon induces intraluminal thrombosis and shrinkage.[23]

Acknowledgements

Figure 2.2(a) is copyright of Steven Newman and is reproduced with permission from Feldon SE. Visual fields in retinal disease. In: Ryan SJ (ed.) *Retina*, vol. 1, ch. 13. St Louis: Mosby, 1989. Figure 2.2(b) is after Anderson DR. *Testing the field of vision.* St Louis: Mosby, 1982. Figures 2.8 and 2.9 are reproduced from Holder GE. *J Neurol Neurosurg Psychiatry* 1989;52:1364–9.

1 Ferris FL III, Sperduto RD. Standardised illumination for visual acuity testing in clinical research. *Am J Ophthalmol* 1982;94:97–8.
2 Ferris FL III, Kassof KA, Brenick GH, Bailey I. New visual acuity charts for clinical research. *Am J Ophthalmol* 1982;94:91–6.
3 Wetherill JR. Visual acuity assessment. *Eye* 1993;7:26–9.
4 Arden GB. Testing contrast sensitivity in clinical practice. *Clin Vis Sci* 1988;2:213–24.
5 Hart WM. Acquired dyschromatopsias. *Surv Ophthalmol* 1987;32:10–31.
6 Searle AET, Wild JM, Shaw DE, O'Neill EC. Time-related variation in normal automated static perimetry. *Ophthalmology* 1991;98:701–7.
7 Safran AB, Glaser JS. Stato-kinetic dissociation in lesions of the anterior visual pathways. *Arch Ophthalmol* 1980;98:291–5.
8 International Standardisation Committee of the International Society for the Clinical Electrophysiology of Vision. Standard for clinical electroretinography. *Arch Ophthalmol* 1989;107:816–19.
9 Holder GE. Significance of abnormal pattern electroretinography in anterior visual pathway dysfunction. *Br J Ophthalmol* 1987;71:166–71.
10 Kriss A, Russell-Eggitt I. Electrophysiological assessment of visual pathway function in infants. *Eye* 1992;6:145–53.
11 Plant G, Hess R, Thomas S. The pattern evoked electroretinogram in optic neuritis. A combined psychophysical and electrophysiological study. *Brain* 1986;109:469–90.
12 Atta HR. Imaging of the optic nerve with standard echography. *Eye* 1988;2:358–66.
13 Steinke W, Kloetzsch C, Hennerici M. Carotid artery disease assessed by color Doppler imaging: correlation with standard Doppler sonography and angiography. *AJNR* 1990;11:259–66.
14 Spector RH. Echographic diagnosis of dural carotid-cavernous sinus fistulas. *Am J Ophthalmol* 1991;111:77–83.
15 Ho AC, Lieb WE, Flaharty PM, Sergott RC, Brown GC, Bosley TM, Savino PJ. Color Doppler imaging of ocular ischaemic syndrome. *Ophthalmology* 1992;99:1453–62.
16 Williamson TH, Baxter GM, Dutton GN. Colour Doppler velocimetry of the arterial vasculature of the optic nerve head and orbit. *Eye* 1993;7:74–80.
17 Anderson ML. Imaging advances in neuro-ophthalmology. *Curr Opin Ophthalmol* 1992;3:615–19.

18 Lindblom B, Truwit CL, Hoyt WF. Optic nerve sheath meningioma. Definition of intraorbital, intracanalicular and intracranial components with magnetic resonance imaging. *Ophthalmology* 1992;**99**:560–6.

19 Imes RK, Hoyt WF. Magnetic resonance imaging of optic gliomas in neurofibromatosis I. *Am J Ophthalmol* 1991;**111**:729–34.

20 Guy J, Moa J, Bidgood D, Mancuso A, Quisling RG. Enhancement and demyelination of the intraorbital optic nerve on fat suppression magnetic resonance imaging. *Ophthalmology* 1992;**99**:713–19.

21 Hamed LM, Silberger J, Silberger M *et al*. Magnetic resonance angiography of vascular lesions causing neuro-ophthalmic defects. *Surv Ophthalmol* 1993;**37**:425–34.

22 Kwan E, Hieshima GB, Higashida RT, Halbach VV, Wolpert SM. Interventional neuroradiology in neuro-ophthalmology. *J Clin Neuro-Ophthalmol* 1989;**9**:83–97.

23 Brosnahan D, McFadzean RM, Teasdale E. Neuro-ophthalmic features of carotid cavernous fistulas and their treatment by endoarterial balloon embolisation. *J Neurol Neurosurg Psychiatry* 1992; **55**:553–6.

3: Retinal disorders in neuro-ophthalmology

JF ACHESON

3.1 Retinal degeneration in neurodegenerative disease
3.2 Inflammatory diseases of the eye and brain (uveomeningeal syndromes)
3.3 Phakomatoses in neuro-ophthalmology
3.4 Vascular disease of the eye and brain

3.1 Retinal degeneration in neurodegenerative disease

Heredo-familial retinal diseases (dystrophies) and a number of other retinal degenerations frequently present to the ophthalmologist, but may in additon have neurological abnormalities beyond any visual deficit. In other cases, neurological diagnosis may be elusive until an ophthalmic examination supports or rules out an associated retinal disorder. Associated neurological conditions include the mitochondrial cytopathies and chromosomal DNA mutations causing abetalipoproteinaemia, Refsum's disease, Bardet–Biedel syndrome, and Usher's syndrome.

In typical "retinitis pigmentosa" the clinical picture is of bilateral symmetrical chronic progressive visual failure with constricted fields, waxy disc pallor (often with hyaline bodies or disc drusen), attenuated retinal arteries and "bone spicules" of abnormal pigment deposits in the peripheral fundus. The visual fields may be reduced to a 5 degree arc tunnel with preserved central acuity as rod photoreceptors are destroyed while the cones at the fovea are relatively preserved. Such patients will be especially incapacitated in scotopic conditions (night-blindness).[1]

Atypical pigmentary retinopathies include cone and cone–rod dystrophies in which central macular, colour, and high acuity vision are destroyed, first giving rise to central scotomata, nystagmus and

Table 3.1 Typical patterns of retinal involvement in selected neurodegenerative syndromes

Typical retinitis pigmentosa	Abetalipoproteinaemia (Bassen–Kornsweig disease) Adult and infantile Refsum's disease Adrenoleucodystrophy
"Salt-and-pepper" retinopathy without typical bone spicules	Kearnes–Sayre syndrome Usher's syndrome Hallevorden–Spatz disease Myotonic dystrophy Arteriohepatic dysplasia (Alagille's syndrome)
Cone–rod dystrophy with predominantly central acuity loss	Olivocerebellopontine degeneration type III Harding type 2 autosomal dominant spinocerebellar degeneration Bardet–Biedel syndrome Juvenile Batten's disease
Cherry-red spot or other macular abnormalities	Tay–Sachs disease (Gm2 gangliosidase deficiency type 1) Niemann–Pick disease

a bull's eye macular appearance. In other instances, pigmented spicules are absent and there is diffuse mottling of the retinal pigment epithelium together with vascular attenuation ("salt and pepper retinopathy"). In some cases, the retina may appear to be virtually normal in spite of severe loss of function. Detailed electrophysiological testing, fluorescein angiography, and genetic assessment is often invaluable.

Mitochondrial cytopathies

Patients with major deletions of the mitochondrial genome may have pigmentary retinopathy – usually with a salt and pepper pattern (atypical retinitis pigmentosa). The Kearnes–Sayre–(Daroff) syndrome is a subset of chronic progressive ophthalmoplegia (CPEO) with onset before age 20 years, progressive ophthalmoplegia, retinal degeneration and at least one of the following: cardiac conduction abnormalities, elevated CSF protein, or cerebellar dysfunction.[2] In the majority of cases, family members are not affected and mitochondrial DNA deletions are not found in muscle biopsies of the proband's parents. In such sporadic cases the deletion is likely to occur during embryogenesis.

Table 3.2   Differential diagnosis of retinitis pigmentosa

Inflammatory conditions
   Intrauterine infection with rubella, CMV, syphilis

Toxic
   Thioridazine
   Chlorpromazine
   Chloroquine
   Tamoxifen

Uniocular
   Trauma
   Diffuse unilateral subacute neuroretinitis (DUSN)

Paraneoplastic retinopathies
   Cancer associated retinopathy
   Melanoma associated retinopathy

Specific idiopathic retinal degenerations
   Acute zonal occult outer retinopathy (AZOOR)
   Big blindspot syndrome
   Multiple evanescent white dot syndrome (MEWDS)

Paraneoplastic retinal degenerations

The chief symptomatic complaint in *cancer-associated retinopathy* (CAR) is of bizarre entoptic phenomena – intermittent spontaneous shimmering lights, floaters or flashing lights, together with declining vision and field defects.[3] Typically a ring scotoma develops from arcuate defects and fundoscopy shows conspicuous retinal arterial narrowing. The ERG is often helpful, and an autoimmune pathogenesis based on the presence of antiphotoreceptor antibodies has been implicated. The search for infective and toxic aetiologies is negative and within a few months remote cancer is discovered.

Many cases are associated with malignant melanoma, when the term *melanoma-associated retinopathy* (MAR) is used.[4]

3.2   Inflammatory diseases of the eye and brain (uveomeningeal syndromes)

The uveomeningeal syndromes are a range of diseases with shared involvement of retina, uveal tract, and brain. In some cases the presentation may be with major neurological abnormalities and the ocular features are asymptomatic and are only discovered on careful examination after pupillary dilatation; in others, the presentation may be with visual loss due to uveitis but there is a

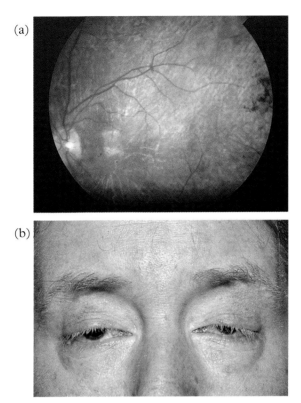

Figure 3.1 Mitochondrial cytopathies and the retina. (a) Retinitis pigmentosa in a patient with mitochondrial cytopathy; (b) ptosis in same patient with mitochondrial cytopathy

relatively asymptomatic CSF pleocytosis. Idiopathic inflammatory disease is the commonest cause of this group of diseases in current UK hospital practice including neurosarcoid, Behçet's disease, the Vogt–Koyanagi–Harada syndrome and systemic vasculitis. Non-Hodgkin's lymphoma is also seen in this context, especially amongst older patients, and tuberculosis, syphilis, and Lyme disease must always be excluded.

Neurosarcoidosis

The eye is involved in 25% of cases of sarcoidosis: hilar adenopathy and lung parenchymal involvement are present in over

49

75%. Extrathoracic disease of skin and joints is frequent but sarcoidosis of the nervous system (neurosarcoid) is relatively uncommon, occurring in only 5% of cases. Neurosarcoid can involve cranial and peripheral nerves, the meninges and brain, and spinal cord parenchyma, resulting in mixed combinations of peripheral and cranial neuropathies, encephalopathy, meningitis, and seizures. Involvement of the visual pathways can cause visual acuity loss, field defects, and diabetes insipidis. Anterior pituitary insufficiency and hypothalamic syndromes also can occur. Twenty per cent of cases of posterior uveitis due to sarcoidosis are associated with CNS disease.

Active ocular disease in the presence of undiagnosed systemic involvement is common and is the presenting mode in 20% of all cases. Anterior uveitis (typically acute granulomatous iritis) arises most commonly, but 30% of ocular sarcoid is confined to the posterior ocular segment. The vitreous, choroid, and optic nerve can all be involved by granulomatous infiltration and the retina shows characteristic periphlebitis (vasculitis).[5,6]

Behçet's disease

In Behçet's disease the protean manifestations include ocular, neurological and systemic features. Ocular involvement occurs in 70–85% of patients, including iridocyclitis with hypopyon, focal retinitis, retinal vein occlusions with vasculitis, and ischaemic optic neuropathy. Neurological features include meningoencephalitis with CSF pleocytosis, dural sinus thrombosis, and focal lesions of cortex, cerebellum, and brain stem. Systemic Behçet's classically consists of orogenital ulceration, arthritis, and dermatoses together with superficial and deep venous thrombosis.[7]

Vogt–Koyanagi–Harada syndrome

The Vogt–Koyanagi–Harada syndrome comprises a panuveitis with neurological and dermatological abnormalities. The ocular abnormalities typically include serious retinal detachment and small creamy-white peripheral fundal lesions together with inflammatory cells in the anterior chamber and vitreous. Neurological changes include symptoms of meningeal inflammation, CSF pleocytosis, cranial neuropathies and specific features of VIIIth nerve involvement (dysacusis and tinnitus). Changes in the skin include poliosis, vitiligo, and alopecia.[8]

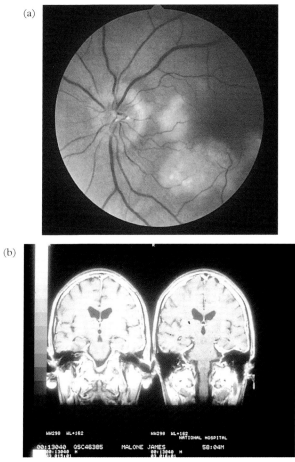

Figure 3.2 (a) Subretinal inflammatory infiltrates and (b) diffuse high meningeal signal on a coronal T-1 weighted MRI scan indicating meningeal inflammation in a patient with a uveomeningeal syndrome due to systemic p-ANCA vasculitis. (Courtesy of Dr EM Graham)

3.3 Phakomatoses in neuro-ophthalmology

Neurofibromatosis types 1 and 2

It is now recognised that although they have overlapping features, including a propensity to neurofibromas and tumours of the central nervous system, NF1 and NF2 are separate diseases

51

which map to separate chromosomes – 17 for NF1 and 22 for NF2. Developmental hamartomas arise in both types.

Neurofibromatosis 1

NF1 is the commonest, with a frequency of about 1 in 3000. The gene has 100% penetrance but variable expression. NF1 is inherited as an autosomal dominant trait but about 50% of new cases are considered to be new mutations. The diagnostic criteria for NF1 are met if a person has two or more of the following:

- Six or more café-au-lait spots over 5 mm in greatest diameter in prepubertal individuals and 15 mm in postpubertal individuals.
- Two or more neurofibromas or one plexiform neuroma.
- Axillary or inguinal freckles.
- Optic glioma.
- Two or more Lisch nodules.
- Distinctive osseous lesion (eg sphenoid dysplasia).
- A first degree relative with NF1.

Ocular features of NF1 include iris hamartomas – Lisch nodules or melanocytic naevi which are detectable in about 50% of 5-year-olds, 75% of 15-year-olds, and 95–100% of adults over 25 years. Individuals with NF1 may also have congenital glaucoma, anterior subcapsular cataract, posterior segment hamartomas, retinal vascular occlusions and pulsating exophthalmos due to sphenoid dysplasia. Retinal and choroidal hamartomas are occasionally seen, but these are a more typical feature of NF2. The gene for NF1 is located on the long arm of chromosome 17 – band q11.2. Within this gene is an area coding for a GAP-like protein which may act as a growth regulator, interacting with an oncogene to produce benign and occasionally malignant tumours. The unpredictability of disease severity even in the same NF1 gene mutation makes genetic counselling exceedingly difficult.[9,10]

Neurofibromatosis 2

Neurofibromatosis 2 is a much rarer disease than NF1, with a population incidence of 1 in 33 000 to 1 in 40 000. At least 50% of new cases appear to be new mutations. Like NF1, NF2 has an extremely high penetrance. The hallmark of NF2 is the presence of bilateral vestibular nerve schwannomas: diagnostic criteria are met if a person has either of the following:

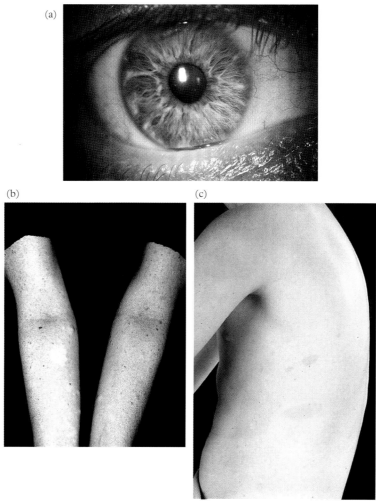

Figure 3.3 Neurofibromatosis type 1 (NF1). (a) Iris Lisch nodules in a patient with NF1; (b) subcutaneous neuromas in NF1; (c) café-au-lait spot in a patient with NF1.

- Bilateral VIIIth nerve masses seen with appropriate imaging.
- A first degree relative with NF2 and either unilateral VIIIth nerve mass or one of the following:
  neurofibromas
  meningioma
  glioma
  schwannoma
  juvenile posterior subcapsular lenticular opacity.

53

Patients with NF2 tend to develop tumours of neural coverings and sheaths – meningiomas, including optic nerve sheath meningiomas, schwannomas, ependymomas – whereas those with NF1 tend to develop neural or astrocytic tumours – astrocytomas and gliomas. Although presentation is typically the result of hearing loss, more than 75% of patients with NF2 have premature visual loss as a result of cataract, and occasionally optic nerve sheath meningioma. Other ocular findings include combined retinal pigment epithelial and retinal hamartomas, epiretinal membranes, optic disc gliomas, retinal haemangiomas, medullated nerve fibres, choroidal naevi, uveal melanoma, and choroidal hamartoma.[11]

In sporadic forms of the disease the vestibular schwannomas develop at a later age and may occur unilaterally.

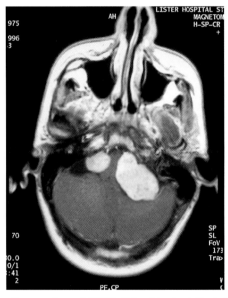

Figure 3.4   Neurofibromatosis type 2 (NF2): T-2 weighted axial brain MRI scan showing bilateral vestibular schwannomas in NF2.

Von Hippel–Lindau disease

Von Hippel–Lindau (VHL) disease is a pleiotrophic autosomal dominant inherited familial cancer syndrome characterised by a predisposition to develop haemangioblastomas of CNS and retina, renal cell carcinoma, phaeochromocytoma, and renal, pancreatic and epididymal cysts. The minimum birth incidence in the United Kingdom is 1 in 36 000. The gene for VHL disease has been mapped to chromosome 3p25–p26, and the clinical importance lies in the fact that long term morbidity and mortality can be reduced by presymptomatic diagnosis of ocular, CNS, and renal involvement.[12]

Although clinical heterogeneity is common, retinal angiomatosis is the most frequent initial manifestation and develops in more than 70% of patients by the age of 60 years. Retinal haemangiomas (or more correctly, haemangioblastomas) are most commonly seen in the peripheral retina but may also occur on the optic disc and at the ora serrata. Ophthalmological screening requires dilated direct and indirect fundoscopy together with fluorescein angioscopy for the detection of nascent, preclinical lesions.[13]

Current criteria for diagnosis are:

1 *No family history*:
   Two of the following features: retinal or CNS haemangio-blastoma, phaeochromocytoma, renal cell carcinoma, or renal/pancreatic/epididymal cysts.
2 *Positive family history*:
   One of the above.

Current screening recommendations in an affected individual are:

1 Annual physical examination and urinalysis, including vanillyl mandelic acid (VMAs).
2 Annual ophthalmological examinations.
3 Brain imaging 3 yearly to age 50, then 5 yearly.
4 Annual renal ultrasound and 3 yearly abdominal CT scanning.

When screening of an at-risk relative is required, this protocol is modified so that the eyes are examined from age of 5 years (with fluorescein angioscopy from age 10), brain imaging is undertaken 3 yearly from age 15 to 40 and then 5 yearly, and abdominal imaging is commenced from age 20.[14]

Tuberose sclerosis complex

The triad of epilepsy, retinal tumours, and adenoma sebaceum, referred to as tuberose sclerosis or Bourneville's disease, has now

(a)

(b)

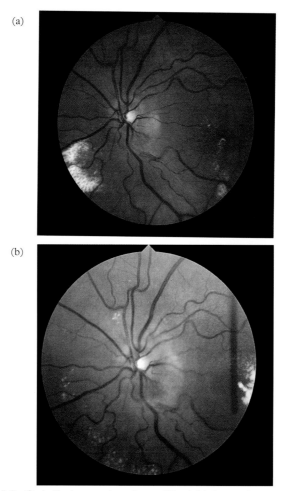

Figure 3.5 Optic disc haemangioma in von Hippel–Lindau syndrome (VHL). (a) At presentation (note peripapillary hard exudate); (b) one year later (note hard exudate at macula); (c) 10 years later (note extensive posterior exudative retinal detachment); (d) total retinal detachment complicating original disc haemangioma; (e) asymptomatic peripheral retinal haemangioma in the fellow eye; (f) asymptomatic peripheral retinal haemangioma in the fellow eye.–continued opposite

been widened and the term tuberose sclerosis complex (TSC) is applied. All tissues are involved, most typically brain and retina but also skin, heart, kidneys and lungs. TSC is inherited as an autosomal dominant trait showing marked genetic heterogeneity.

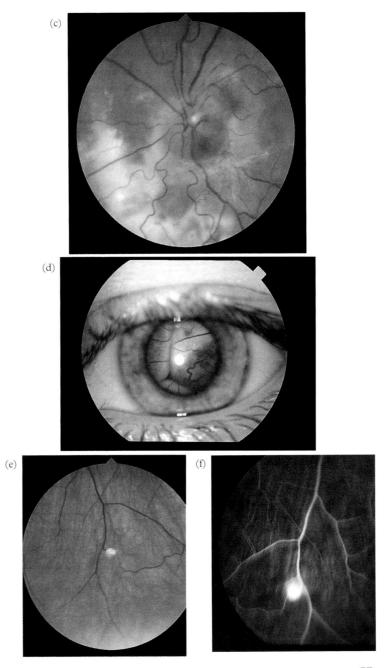

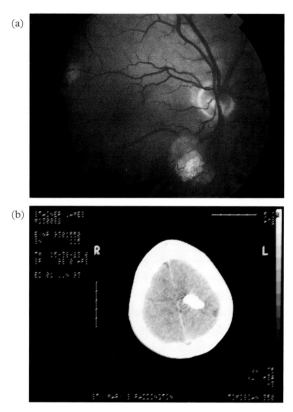

Figure 3.6   Tuberose sclerosis. (a) Calcified (below disc) and non-calcified astrocytic hamartomas in tuberose sclerosis; (b) axial CT brain scan of same patient showing large calcified intracranial hamartoma; (c) (opposite) optic disc astrocytic hamartoma in tuberose sclerosis: in contrast to disc haemangiomas, progressive visual loss is not typical.

Fifty per cent of patients have retinal or optic nerve hamartomas: other ocular abnormalities include adenoma sebaceum on the eyelids and colobomas. A wide range of neuro-ophthalmic features including retrochiasmal field defects, ocular motility abnormalities, and papilloedema reflect intracranial involvement. The retinal hamartomas may be calcified or non-calcified lesions of both glioblastic and angioblastic origin – patches of focal congenital retinal pigment epithelial hypertrophy may also be seen. In contrast to von Hippel-Lindau disease, retinal hamartomas in TSC are only rarely associated with visual loss.[15]

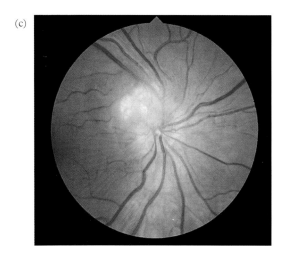

Sturge–Weber syndrome (encephalo-trigeminal angiomatosis)

Sturge–Weber syndrome is a further vascular neurocutaneous syndrome classed with the phakomatoses, but which, unlike VHL disease, does not appear to have a familial basis. Facial cavernous angiomas are commonly found in the distribution of the ophthalmic division of the trigeminal nerve. Intracranial calcifying occipitoparietal leptomeningeal angiomata on the same side as the facial lesion result in underlying cortical abnormalities with epilepsy, homonymous hemianopia and, in some cases, mental retardation. Ipsilateral ocular involvement is characteristic, with glaucoma and hae-mangiomas of choroid, conjunctiva and episclera arising in over half of all cases. In other patients, asymptomatic retinal vascular tortuosity and iris heterochromia have been noted. Some patients have isolated facial or intracranial lesions.[16]

3.4   Vascular disease of the eye and brain

Retinal transient ischaemic attacks (TIAs) and strokes

Transient monocular blindness (amaurosis fugax) and acute monocular visual failure are usually the result of temporary or permanent occlusion of the central or branch retinal arteries, or of the blood supply to the optic nerve head.

Transient monocular blindness

The term transient monocular blindness is used to cover a variety of symptoms. These include typical amaurosis fugax in which the patient reports the drawing of a black veil across the visual field from above or below to extinguish vision either completely or in a hemifield and lasting for a period of 1–5 minutes. Complete recovery follows in about 15–20 minutes with gradual clearing in a reverse direction. This history is strongly suggestive of the passage of an embolism across the retinal circulation, resulting in an initial proximal occlusion of either the central retinal artery or one of its main branches before breaking up and dispersing into the periphery. The differential diagnosis of transient visual loss becomes much narrower if these details can be elicited – in particular the monocular nature and the time course. By contrast, transient visual loss due to raised intracranial pressure with papilloedema is typically very fleeting, with momentary monocular or binocular fading of vision on coughing, Valsalva manoeuvre or sudden postural change. Sometimes benign orbital tumours present with gaze evoked amaurosis in which vision is lost only when the eye turns in a particular direction as a result of intraorbital ophthalmic artery compression. Stuttering visual loss in which field or acuity fade, partially recover and then fade again suggests the onset of ischaemic optic neuropathy, whilst a more sustained gradual fading of vision, particularly after exposure to bright light with positive visual phenomena, is indicative of retinal ischaemia arising from chronic hypoperfusion.

Central retinal artery (CRA) occlusion

Sudden painless blindness is the presenting symptom of a central retinal artery occlusion unless a cilioretinal artery is present to supply blood to the macula. Examination of the pupils confirms a relative afferent pupil defect, and the ophthalmoscopic appearances depend upon how soon after the onset of symptoms the examination is performed. In the first few minutes "cattle-truck" segmentation of the venous blood column is seen with arterial attenuation. Mild digital pressure on the globe will induce segmentation of the arterial blood column confirming slow circulation. In ophthalmic artery occlusion the intraocular pressure is reduced. After an hour or so the ischaemic retina develops a white appearance with a cherry-red spot at the fovea due to the normal red colour of the choroid showing through where the neurosensory retina is absent. Within

Table 3.3   Conditions associated with transient monocular blindness

Intraocular
  Glaucoma (intermittent angle closure causing corneal oedema)
  Anterior ischaemic optic neuropathy
Intraorbital (mass effect causing gaze evoked amaurosis)
  Haemangioma
  Meningioma
Intracranial
  Raised intracranial pressure (visual obscurations)
Carotid artery
  Thromboembolism
  Stenosis and occlusion
    arteritis
    fibromuscular dysplasia
    dissecting aneurysm
    radiation angiopathy
Cardiac
  Valvular emboli
    calcific aortic stenosis
    endocarditis
    mitral valve prolapse
  Mural thrombosis
    cardiac dysrhythmias
    post infarction
  Atrial myxoma
Miscellaneous
  Migraine
  Paradoxical embolism

a few days the cherry-red spot and retinal opacification disappears leaving optic atrophy and retinal artery attenuation.

Amaurosis fugax as a premonitory symptom of CRA suggests an embolic cause. In patients under 40 years, the heart is the commonest source, due to rheumatic valve disease, mitral valve

Five causes of central retinal artery occlusion

- Embolic obstruction
- Occlusion in situ in association with atheroma with superimposed thrombosis or haemorrhage
- Inflammatory arteritis, eg temporal arteritis, polyarteritis nodosa, thromboangiitis obliterans
- Simple vasospasm, eg in Raynaud's disease or migraine
- Arterial occlusion secondary to low perfusion pressure in carotid stenosis, aortic arch syndrome or traumatic globe compression

prolapse, endocarditis, or atrial myxoma and careful cardiological assessment is essential. When standard echocardiography is negative, a transoesophageal study may be helpful. In older patients the source may be cardiac or arterial from atheromatous ulceration of the aorta or ipsilateral internal carotid artery.

The differential diagnosis of CRA includes acute ischaemic optic neuropathy (AION), acute central retinal vein occlusion, retinal detachment, vitreous haemorrhage, and non-organic (functional) visual loss. Although irreversible damage to the retina occurs after 2 hours at the most, prompt initial treatment may help to restore at least some degree of vision. This should include ocular massage to lower the intraocular pressure and help dislodge an embolus into the peripheral retinal circulation, and intravenous Diamox. Heparin anticoagulation may be helpful in impending CRA occlusion and high dose corticosteroids are indicated if giant cell arteritis is suspected.[17,18]

Branch retinal artery (BRA) occlusion

The lodging of an embolus at a first or second order bifurcation of the central retinal artery results in a branch retinal artery occlusion, producing an area of pallid retinal oedema and sudden and permanent loss of the corresponding visual field. Emboli can often be seen in the fundus: the commonest form is the fibrin-platelet Hollenhorst plaque derived from an ulcerated atheromatous carotid artery plaque. Other materials include calcific deposits from a cardiac valve or atheromatous plaque, amniotic fluid, fat in pancreatitis and long bone fractures, and foreign bodies such a talc in intravenous drug abusers. Sometimes asymptomatic emboli are discovered: these patients should be treated as though they were at the same risk of stroke as those with visual loss.

Reducing the risk of cerebral hemisphere stroke in CRA and BRA

To reduce the risk of stroke all patients are evaluated for associated hypertension, cardiac disease, arterial vascular disease, and the presence of antiphospholipid antibodies. A carotid bruit may be heard, but its absence does not necessarily mean normal vessels.

Doppler ultrasonography of the carotid bifurcation is widely used and together with Duplex imaging of the lumen and plaque dimensions provides useful non-invasive data on the degree of stenosis, the presence of calcification and ulceration, and haemo-dynamic abnormalities across the stenotic lesion. Intravenous digital subtraction angiography and magnetic resonance angiography provide alternatives to direct arterial puncture techniques with less morbidity and less resolution. Only those patients with a stenosis occluding between 70 and 99% of the vascular lumen are significantly less likely to develop a cerebral hemisphere stroke if they undergo endarterectomy as opposed to optimal medical management with antiplatelet agents. Patients with symptomatic carotid stenosis of less than 30% do not appear to benefit from surgery and do just as well with optimal medical therapy (careful management of hypertension and use of antiplatelet agents). The selection of patients for endarterectomy must also depend on the assessment of risk of death from coronary artery disease which usually is also present, and on the morbidity and mortality of angiography and surgery at the centre offering treatment. In practice only a minority of patients who present with retinal transient ischaemic attacks (amaurosis fugax), retinal strokes (artery occlusions) or cerebral hemisphere TIAs will definitely be helped by endarterectomy.[19–21]

Giant cell arteritis (see also Chapter 9)

Giant cell (cranial or temporal) arteritis is a systemic disorder featuring an inflammatory arteritis of medium sized, elastin containing vessels, particularly involving the extradural branches of the external and internal carotid arteries. The most prominent clinical feature is headache. This is felt in the scalp, usually in the territory of inflamed vessels along the course of the superficial temporal and occipital arteries and their branches. The patient may notice localised swelling and redness in these areas. Palpation may confirm redness and localised oedema with loss of pulsation and tenderness. Many patients complain spontaneously of scalp tenderness, such as when resting their head on the pillow, or on brushing or combing hair. In addition, there may be muscular ache affecting the hips and shoulder (polymyalgia rheumatica) which may precede the onset of headache by a period of several months. Polymyalgia may be associated with weight loss, sweating, and low grade pyrexia. Jaw claudication may also be reported where there is pain on mastication which is relieved on resting.

Involvement of the ophthalmic artery leads to visual loss from ischaemic optic neuropathy (see Chapter 4) often combined with a central retinal artery occlusion. Cranial arteritis is also a cause of amaurosis fugax. Visual loss may be posturally dependent with

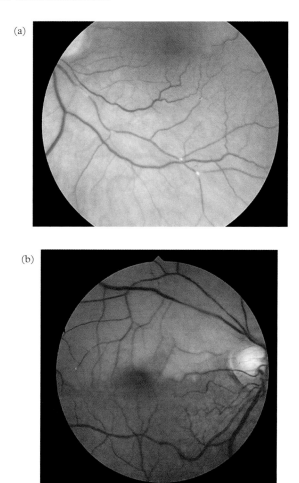

Figure 3.7 Retinal artery occlusions. (a) Multiple retinal cholesterol emboli in a patient with amaurosis fugax; (b) single peripheral retinal cholesterol embolus in a patient with an inferior branch retinal artery occlusion causing a sectoral retinal infarct; (c) central retinal artery occlusion in a patient without visible emboli: the underlying diagnosis was antiphospholipid antibody syndrome complicating systemic lupus erythematosus; (d) slow flow retinopathy; (e) proliferative retinopathy and vitreous haemorrhage in a non-diabetic patient with extracranial carotid artery occlusions. – continued opposite

symptoms on standing or sitting up which are relieved on lying down. Occasionally visual loss may occur in the absence of headache. Less commonly, vertebrobasilar ischaemia may be

(c)

(d)

(e)

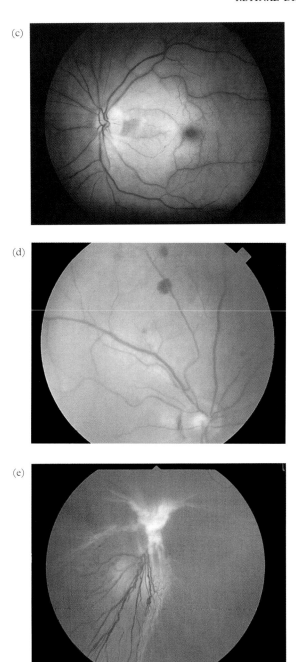

prominent, and there may be an external ophthalmoplegia as a result of involvement of the extraocular muscles or the intraorbital portion of the ocular motor nerves (III, IV and VI) or both. As a general rule the intracranial arteries are spared; however, cerebral or brain stem infarction may result from complete inflammatory occlusion of the extracranial vessels or from embolism from mural thrombus in inflamed arteries.[22] Cranial arteritis is a systemic disease and in some patients the granulomatous arteritis produces prominent vascular occlusion away from the head and neck, involving the aortic arch, or subclavian and coronary vessels, or causing mononeuritis multiplex.

In addition to a normochromic normocytic anaemia, the ESR is regularly and markedly elevated in 90% of untreated patients with established disease. Acute phase proteins (C-reactive protein, fibrinogen, alpha$_2$ and gamma globulins) are also elevated. Autoantibodies are negative. Histology shows a subacute granulomatous arteritis with thickening of the vessel wall and occasional obliteration of the lumen. Because up to 10% of patients may have an ESR of less than 40 mm/h, biopsy is indicated in most cases.[23] Foreign body giant cells are found in relation to focal necrosis of the media and elastic lamina. However, false negative biopsies also arise in up to one-third of cases because of the presence of skip lesions and serial sections of a long (2 cm) length of artery should be undertaken to maximise the chances of histological confirmation of the diagnosis. In the orbit, the arteritis may involve the main trunk and all the branches of the ophthalmic artery including the short posterior ciliary vessels and the central retinal artery within the dural sheath. Arteries within the optic nerve and retina are spared.

Steroids are started immediately on suspicion of the diagnosis, without awaiting the result of a biopsy. Nevertheless, because the management of the condition may extend over many years, histological confirmation is invaluable. Biopsy is best performed within 48 hours of initiating steroid treatment. Following the introduction of steroids (oral prednisolone 60–80 mg daily, or IV methyl prednisolone 500 mg–1 g daily for 3 days), relief of head-ache, malaise, and polymyalgia is usually dramatic. Salvage of vision in established optic nerve or retinal ischaemia is exceptional, but general supportive measures such as lowering the intraocular pressure to improve optic nerve head perfusion, and lying the patient down in bed may help. Low doses of subcutaneous heparin can also be used when there is second eye involvement at presentation. Over the following weeks and months a tapering dose of steroids is then given, titrated against the clinical symptoms and the ESR.

Venous stasis retinopathy and chronic ocular ischaemia

Chronic severe ocular ischaemia may produce a constellation of symptoms, beginning initially with venous stasis retinopathy in the posterior pole and progressing to anterior segment abnormalities.

The retinal changes are not specific to carotid disease and may also be seen in patients with other disease processes which interfere with the oxygen carrying capacity of blood in the retinal circulation, such as blood dyscrasia, hyperviscosity syndromes, and severe anaemia. The patient may complain of mild to severe blurring of vision and of dazzling in bright light which may reflect photoreceptor hypoxia. Diabetic retinopathy and central retinal vein occlusion may share overlapping features reflecting the common retinal response to ischaemia: however, in slow flow retinopathy marked asymmetry in retinal involvement is frequent and large blot haemorrhages may be prominent, and in central retinal vein occlusion conspicuous haemorrhages and nerve fibre layer infarcts (cotton wool spots) cause a "blood and thunder retina".[24,25]

Carotid–cavernous sinus fistulas

When communications arise between the carotid artery and the venous circulation in the region of the cavernous sinus the venous pressure in the globe and orbit rises and the arterial perfusion pressure of the globe may fall, resulting in abnormalities of both vision and eye movements. Fistulas may be classified as:

- Direct/indirect
- Traumatic/spontaneous
- High flow/low flow
- Anatomical configuration on angiography:
    Type A: Intracavernous carotid artery – cavernous sinus
    Type B: Extradural branches of internal carotid – cavernous sinus
    Type C: Extradural branches of external carotid – cavernous sinus

Type D: Extradural branches of both internal and external carotid – cavernous sinus

(Most commonly, direct fistulas (type A) have a high flow and indirect (types B–D) have low flow.)

Table 3.4   Ocular findings with venous stasis retinopathy and ischaemic oculopathy

---

Venous stasis retinopathy
  dot and blot retinal haemorrhages
  microaneurysms
  venous congestion
  irregular calibre of retinal veins
  neovascularisation
  macular oedema
  mild disc swelling

Diffuse oculopathy
  iris/angle neovascularisation
  intraocular pressure change
  corneal oedema
  uveitis
  sluggish pupillary light reactions
  episcleral vascular congestion

Direct carotid–cavernous fistulas

Direct fistulas may be located anywhere along the course of the intracavernous carotid artery and may project anteriorly or posteriorly. The commonest cause is head trauma which may be either penetrating or non-penetrating, and is not necessarily associated with basal skull fracture. Symptoms may not develop for days or weeks after the initial injury. Sometimes a fistula results from spontaneous rupture of a pre-existing aneurysm of the intracavernous carotid artery which may previously have been asymptomatic. Less commonly they arise spontaneously against a background of systemic vasculopathy such as arteriosclerosis and hypertension or fibromuscular dysplasia.

Clinical features   If blood escapes posteriorly through the superior and inferior petrosal sinuses the ocular signs may be minimal, although a lateral rectus palsy is frequently seen as the VIth nerve is compressed by an expanded inferior petrosal sinus. Anterior redirection of arterial blood through normal orbital venous channels leads to ocular manifestations due to raised episcleral venous pressure, reduced arterial perfusion pressure, and venous stasis. The eye involved is not always ipsilateral to the site of the fistula as there are variable connections between the two cavernous sinuses and bilateral ocular signs may arise from the same lesion. Proptosis is typically pulsatile with associated chemosis and arterialisation of the conjunctival vessels. A bruit may be heard by the patient or may only be detected on auscultation. When pulsation and a bruit are absent, the diagnosis is strongly suggested by a wide pulse pressure on applanation tonometry.

Diplopia is common: this is a result of a number of mechanisms acting either in isolation or in combination. First, in trauma patients the ocular motor nerves may be damaged by a basal skull fracture. Secondly, the nerves may be compressed by expansion of the cavernous or inferior petrosal sinus or become hypoxic due to alterations of blood flow in the vasa nervorum. Most commonly the abducens nerve is involved, probably because of its location within the cavernous sinus. Thirdly, orbital hypoxia and oedema with venous stasis results in ophthalmoplegia due to direct myopathic effects. By the same mechanisms the pupil may be abnormal due to intraocular hypoxia or as a result of damage to sympathetic and parasympathetic fibres.

Visual loss is also common in patients with direct carotid–cavernous fistula. Sometimes this is the result of ischaemic optic neuropathy, intracranial optic nerve compression or corneal ulceration, but typically is due to retinal ischaemia. This is due to both a reduction in retinal blood flow as a result of a drop in effective ophthalmic artery perfusion pressure together with venous stasis caused by arterialisation of the orbital venous circulation. Ophthalmoscopy reveals features of a slow flow retinopathy with mild disc swelling, blot haemorrahges and microaneurysms, and venous congestion and tortuosity. A picture of full-blown central retinal vein occlusion may develop; other patients have non-rhegmatogenous retinal detachments and vitreous haemorrhage.

A further mechanism for visual loss is glaucoma. This is usually due to raised episcleral venous pressure with a delayed and insidious onset, but neovascular (rubeosis) and ciliary block mechanisms may also apply in a more acute context.[26]

Endovascular interventional radiology offers effective treatment for direct carotid–cavernous fistula in many cases.[27]

Indirect carotid–cavernous fistulas (types B–D)

The indirect carotid–cavernous fistulas are thought generally to arise from congenital arteriovenous anomalies which become symptomatic in later life in association with other vascular disorders such as hypertension and atherosclerosis. With higher flow rates, the clinical picture becomes indistinguishable from a direct fistula.

Between 20 and 50% of dural carotid–cavernous fistulas close spontaneously – and sometimes after angiography. In those with a persistent fistula there may be eventual visual loss due to glaucoma or to retinal vasculopathy. Sometimes the clinical picture of orbital congestion may dramatically worsen but this does not necessarily indicate increased flow and may instead reflect thrombosis of the superior ophthalmic vein, demonstrable on MRI or with colour Doppler flow mapping techniques. Treatment is indicated in selected cases only.[28]

1 Pagon RA. Retinitis pigmentosa. *Surv Ophthalmol* 1988;**33**:137–77.
2 Mullie MA, Harding AE, Petty RKH *et al.* The retinal manifestations of mitochondrial myopathy: a study of 22 cases. *Arch Ophthalmol* 1985; **103**:1825–30.
3 Thirkill CE, Roth AM, Keltner JL. Cancer associated retinopathy. *Arch Ophthalmol* 1987;**105**:372–5.
4 Berson EL, Lessell S. Paraneoplastic night blindness with malignant melanoma. *Am J Ophthalmol* 1988;**106**:307–11.
5 Delaney P. Neurologic manifestations in sarcoidosis: review of the literature, with a report of 23 cases. *Ann Intern Med* 1977;**87**:336–45.
6 Stern BJ, Krumbolz A, Johns C *et al.* Sarcoidosis and its neurologic manifestations. *Arch Neurol* 1985;**42**:909–17.
7 Barnes CG. Behçet's syndrome. *J R Soc Med* 1984;**77**:816–18.
8 Moorthy RS, Inomata H, Rao NA. Vogt–Koyanagi–Harada syndrome. *Surv Ophthalmol* 1995;**39**:265–92.
9 Ragge NK. Clinical and genetic patterns of neurofibromatosis 1 and 2. *Br J Ophthalmol* 1993;**77**:662–72.
10 Gutman DH, Collins FS. Recent progress toward the understanding of the molecular biology of Von Recklinghausen neurofibromatosis. *Ann Neurol* 1992;**31**:555–61.
11 Narod SA, Parry DM, Parboosingh J *et al.* Neurofibromatosis type 2 appears to be a genetically homogeneous disease. *Am J Hum Genet* 1992;**51**:486–96.
12 Richards EM, Maher ER, Latif F *et al.* Detailed mapping of the VHL disease tumour suppressor gene. *J Med Genet* 1993;**30**:104–7.
13 Maher ER, Yates JR, Harries R *et al.* Clinical features and natural history of von Hippel Lindau disease. *Q J Med* 1990;**77**:1151–63.
14 Moore AT, Maher ER, Rosen P, Gregor Z, Bird AC. Ophthalmological screening for von Hippel Lindau disease. *Eye* 1991;**5**:723–8.
15 Zimmer Galler IE, Robertson DM. Tuberose sclerosis: long term observation of retinal lesions in tuberose sclerosis. *Am J Ophthalmol* 1995;**119**:318–24.

16 Sullivan TJ, Clarke MP, Morin JD. The ocular manifestations of Sturge Weber syndrome. *J Paediatr Ophthalmol Strabismus* 1992;**29**: 349–56.

17 Howard RS, Russell RWR. Prognosis of patients with retinal embolism. *J Neurol Neurosurg Psychiatry* 1987;**50**:1142–7.

18 Wray SH. The management of acute visual failure. *J Neurol Neurosurg Psychiatry* 1993;**56**:234–40.

19 Poole CJM, Russell RWR. Mortality and stroke after amaurosis fugax. *J Neurol Neurosurg Psychiatry* 1985;**48**:902–5.

20 European Carotid Surgery Trialist Collaborative Group MRC European Carotid Surgery Trial. Interim results for symptomatic patients with severe (70–99%) or mild (0–29%) carotid stenosis. *Lancet* 1991;**337**:1235–43.

21 North American Symptomatic Carotid Endarterectomy Trial Collaborators. Beneficial effect of carotid endarterectomy in symptomatic patients with high-grade carotid stenosis. *N Engl J Med* 1991;**325**: 445–53.

22 Wilkinson IM, Russell RW. Arteries of the head and neck in giant cell arteritis: a pathological study to show the pattern of arterial involvement. *Arch Neurol* 1972;**27**:378–92.

23 Jacobson DM, Slamovits TL. The ESR and its relationship to haematocrit in giant cell arteritis. *Arch Ophthalmol* 1987;**105**:965–7.

24 Ross-Russell RW, Ikeda H. Clinical and electrophysiological observations in patients with low pressure retinopathy. *Br J Ophthalmol* 1986; **70**:651–6.

25 Russell RWR, Page NGR. Critical perfusion of eye and brain. *Brain* 1983;**106**:419–34.

26 Sanders MD, Hoyt WF. Hypoxic ocular sequelae of carotid–cavernous fistulas: study of the causes of visual failure before and after neurosurgical treatment in a series of 25 cases. *Br J Ophthalmol* 1969;**53**: 82–97.

27 Kupersmith MJ, Berenstein A, Flamm E, Ransohoff J. Neuroophthalmologic abnormalities and intravascular therapy of traumatic carotid–cavernous fistulas. *Ophthalmology* 1986;**93**:906–12.

28 Kupersmith MJ, Berenstein A, Choi IS, Warren F, Flamm E. Management of nontraumatic vascular shunts involving the cavernous sinus. *Ophthalmology* 1988;**95**:121–30.

4: Optic nerve and chiasmal disease

JF ACHESON

4.1 Pathophysiology of optic nerve disease and the swollen optic disc

Pathophysiology of optic nerve disease

Optic disc swelling
The common feature of optic disc swelling from all causes is stasis of both fast and slow retrograde axoplasmic transport. This results in axonal distension which is ophthalmoscopically visible at the level of the prelaminar optic nerve as a swollen disc. The cause of impaired axoplasmic transport varies from disease to disease: in raised intracranial pressure, the intrasheath CSF pressure of the

anterior optic nerve also rises leading to compromise of axonal function at the lamina cribrosa. In ischaemic optic neuropathy, vascular insufficiency of branches of short posterior ciliary vessels which supply the retrolaminar and laminar portions of the optic nerve head leads to axonal damage. In inflammatory optic neuritis, perivascular inflammatory cellular infiltration and interstitial oedema results in axonal compression and disc oedema. As a result of axonal swelling, secondary vascular changes follow which include capillary dilatation, microaneurysms, haemorrhages, and cotton wool spots on the disc and neighbouring retina in the distribution of the long radial peripapillary arteries as well as dilatation and venous stasis of the prelaminar capillaries, and dilatation of the central retinal vein.[1]

Optic atrophy

In optic atrophy, the reduction in the volume of the capillary bed within the neuroretinal tissue of the nerve head accounts for ophthalmoscopic pallor, together with loss of tissue volume and astrocytic proliferation.[2]

Patterns of visual loss in optic nerve disease

The hallmark of visual loss due to acquired optic nerve disease is a central scotoma, because axons serving macular vision appear to be differentially sensitive to disease processes throughout the course of the nerve. Exceptions to this principle have diagnostic implications: an altitudinal field defect suggests a vascular occlusion, a centrocaecal scotoma suggests heredo-familial or toxic damage to the fibres of the foveal and centrocaecal projections in the anterior optic nerve, and a constricted field with preserved acuity suggests either post-papilloedema optic atrophy or a retinal dystrophy. When there is acute loss of function with a normal optic nerve head on fundoscopy, the term retrobulbar optic neuropathy is used. When visual loss is associated with disc swelling, the terms papillitis or papillopathy are often used. Optic atrophy may follow both variants after about 6 weeks.

Differential diagnosis of the swollen optic disc

The terms optic disc swelling and papilloedema are often used interchangeably, irrespective of aetiology. However, current convention reserves the term papilloedema for the syndrome of pathological disc swelling due to raised intracranial pressure. The remainder of cases are designated either as disc swelling arising from a local (ie in the eye or orbit) lesion or as pseudopapill-oedema when the appearance arises as a congenital anomaly. This classification may help the clinician to think clearly when approaching the differential diagnosis.

Disc swelling from local causes

Disc oedema due to local optic nerve disease is normally associated with early loss of acuity and colour vision, together with central, arcuate or altitudinal field defects. Involvement is usually unilateral and consequently there is a relative afferent pupil defect.

Pseudopapilloedema

The appearance of "pseudopapilloedema" mimicking true papilloedema of raised intracranial pressure may cause difficulties. All too frequently the patient with headaches is wrongly thought to have raised intracranial pressure from the fundoscopic finding of elevated discs. A systematic approach is essential to resolve this difficulty:

1   Does the headache have the features of raised pressure (more severe on awakening, exacerbated by coughing)?
2   What is the approximate refraction of the eye? Hypermetropes often have small, crowded, elevated discs which are a normal variant. Similarly, myopes frequently have dysverted or tilted discs with an elevated indistinct margin supernasally.
3   What can be learnt on careful fundoscopy?

In true papilloedema secondary vascular changes are usually prominent with prepapillary capillary dilatation, haemorrhages, and exudates as well as axonal swelling. Spontaneous pulsation of the central retinal vein is not always observed in the normal subject, but when seen, raised intracranial pressure is highly unlikely. Superficial disc drusen appear as refractile bodies on the disc surface causing abnormal elevation, and hamartomas produce a mass effect without these vascular changes. Buried disc drusen result in an indistinct disc margin often with an anomalous retinal vascular pattern with trifurcations of the first order vessels at the disc margin. Sometimes further investigations are required. Intrapapillary calcification of drusen can be seen on CT scanning and ultrasound. Fundus fluorescein angiography shows an absence of any vascular dilatation or late leakage from the prepapillary capillaries: typically, the disc shows late staining with fluorescein but without leakage beyond the disc margins. Buried disc drusen show autofluorescence when illuminated with blue light.[3]

Classification of papilloedema

In papilloedema due to raised intracranial pressure the disc swelling is usually but not always bilateral and symmetrical. Over a period of time, the clinical features evolve through a sequence of stages designated *early, acute, chronic, vintage,* and *atrophic.*

In *early* papilloedema there is simply blurring of the disc margins as axons swell, together with loss of spontaneous venous pulsation.

In the *acute* full-blown picture there are also features of secondary vascular changes with haemorrhages, hard exudates, and cotton wool spots. Symptoms include momentary fading of vision (obscurations) associated with postural changes or on the Valsalva manoeuvre, reflecting vascular compromise. At this point, perimetry shows blindspot enlargement only as swollen axons displace peripapillary photoreceptors. Visual acuity and colour vision remain normal.

In *chronic* papilloedema, compensatory mechanisms lead to the resolution of the vascular abnormalities leaving axonal swelling with signs of mild vascular congestion in the form of dilatation of the prepapillary capillaries.

Later, in *vintage* papilloedema involutional changes can be seen in the form of early disc pallor and the appearance of white refractile bodies on the disc surface – corpora amylacea.

Finally, in *atrophic* papilloedema axonal loss is conspicuous leading to loss of supporting glial and vascular elements and flattening of the disc with retinal vascular attenuation. As a rule, it is only in chronic papilloedema that visual acuity loss is seen, either as a result of axonal loss, or occasionally because of adjacent subretinal neovascularisation.

Visual loss secondary to chronic raised intracranial pressure

The management of chronic raised intracranial pressure depends upon the careful separation of truly idiopathic cases from those in which there is an identifiable cause requiring specific treatment.

(a)

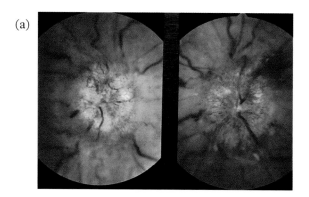

(b)

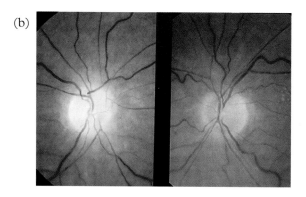

(c)

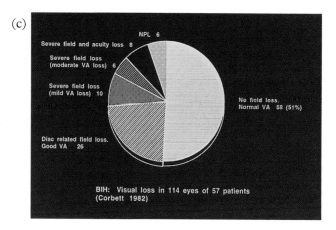

(d)

(e)

(f)

SA 5.11.91

LE
VAL 6/5
N 10

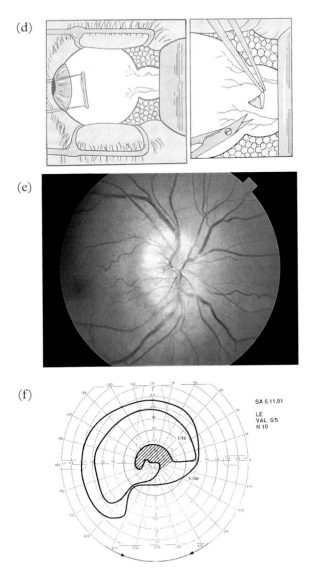

Figure 4.1   Optic disc swelling. (a) Full-blown (decompensated) papilloedema; (b) late atrophic papilloedema; (c) proportion of patients with chronic raised intracranial pressure due to idiopathic intracranial hypertension developing significant levels of visual loss (114 eyes, 57 patients); (d) the technique of optic nerve sheath decompression; (e) swollen optic disc: without information on the acuity, pupillary light reflex, and visual field, it is impossible to guess the cause; (f) visual field in the same patient: an inferior altitudinal defect plus superior arcuate scotoma points towards a diagnosis of ischaemic optic neuropathy.

Idiopathic intracranial hypertension

Whilst idiopathic intracranial hypertension (pseudotumour cerebri, benign intracranial hypertension) may carry a good prognosis for life when compared to many other diseases causing papilloedema, the condition is far from benign in terms of visual function. More than 80% of patients have been shown eventually to develop some degree of visual loss, and up to 10% have significant field defects and acuity loss rather than simply obscurations and blindspot enlargement, and careful follow-up is required.[4] Medical measures to control headache and visual symptoms in chronic raised intracranial pressure may be both ineffective and poorly tolerated. These include weight loss, carbonic anhydrase inhibitors, corticosteroids, and serial lumbar punctures. Surgical CSF diversion procedures may be required and include lumboperitoneal shunting and optic nerve sheath decompression (fenestration).[5,6]

4.2   Developmental abnormalities

Hypoplasia

Hypoplasia of the optic disc may be unilateral or bilateral, obvious or subtle and may be associated with both good and poor visual function. There is a subnormal number of axons within the affected nerve although the mesodermal elements and glial supporting cells are both normal.

The diagnosis is normally made on the basis of marked reduction of disc substance. This typically leaves an area of bare exposed sclera which coincides with a gap between the retinal pigment epithelial border and the true disc margin. The retinal nerve fibre layer is thinned. In less marked cases diagnosis becomes more difficult and photographic methods to evaluate the ratio of the centre disc/ fovea distance to the disc diameter may be valuable: a ratio of more than 3.0 is considered to be diagnostic. Field defects are variable and may reflect more extensive visual pathway anomalies: as a general rule the smaller the disc, the worse the visual acuity.

Optic nerve hypoplasia may occur as an isolated defect or in association with a wide range of facial, ocular, and intracranial anomalies reflecting the embryological derivation from the forebrain. These include albinism, aniridia, ocular colobomas, Duane's syndrome, Klippel–Trenauney–Weber syndrome, Goldenhar syndrome, blepharophimosis, hemifacial atrophy and septo-optic dysplasia (de Morsier's syndrome). More extensive brain malformations are sometimes seen.[7,8]

No single aetiology has been identified but there is an association with the fetal alcohol syndrome and maternal crack cocaine use as well as with phenytoin, LSD, and quinine.

Other congenital disc anomalies

Colobomas and pits

In contrast to optic nerve hypoplasia, optic disc colobomas and pits are thought to arise as a consequence of faulty closure of the embryonic fetal fissure of the optic stalk and cup. Other colobomas involving the lens, iris, and choroid are frequently seen in association. A variety of forms may occur, and each may be associated with acuity loss or field defects: enlarged discs with deep excavation which may be mistaken for glaucomatous cupping; enlarged discs in which the central excavation is filled with embryonic vascular and glial remnants ("morning glory disc"); excavated discs contiguous with retinochoroidal colobomas; and slightly enlarged discs containing pits within the borders of the nerve head.

In addition to being mistaken for glaucoma, two associations are important: first, basal encephalocoeles, which must be considered in the differential diagnosis of masses in the orbit and nasopharynx, and secondly, with serous retinal detachment.

Dysversions, crescents, and situs inversus

Congenital tilted discs arise when the optic nerve enters the globe at an extremely oblique angle and an associated crescent is seen when there is a disparity between the scleral and retinal openings. The term situs inversus describes the apparent origin of the retinal vessels from the temporal side of the disc rather than the nasal: the disc itself may in addition be hypoplastic. This anomaly is important clinically for two reasons: first, the oblique entry of the optic nerve into the globe means that often the inferonasal margin of the disc is deficient with associated retinal nerve fibre layer defects in this quadrant. As a result temporal field defects result and the patient may be erroneously thought to have chiasmal compression. However, in this situation, careful perimetry shows that the temporal field defect is sloping and does not respect

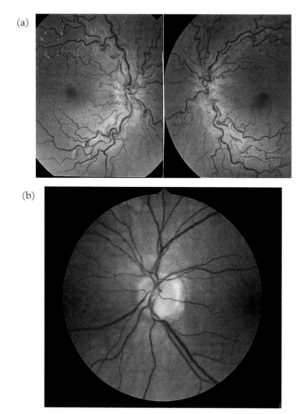

Figure 4.2   Pseudopapilloedema. (a) Crowded hypermetropic discs plus congenital retinal vascular tortuosity; (b) buried optic disc drusen (note absent cup, anomalous vascular pattern, and mild disc elevation); (c) autofluorescent disc drusen; (d) peripapillary telangiectatic microangiopathy in Leber's hereditary optic neuropathy. – continued opposite

the vertical meridian. Secondly, the opposite, healthy side of the disc – usually the superotemporal aspect – is frequently elevated, resulting in the incorrect diagnosis of pathological disc swelling.

4.3   Heredo-familial optic neuropathies

Leber's hereditary optic neuropathy

Leber's hereditary optic neuropathy (LHON) is readily distinguished from other hereditary optic neuropathies by a characteristic clinical presentation: sudden central visual loss in

(c)

(d)

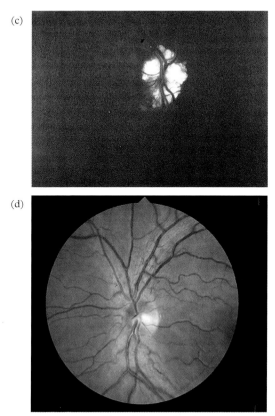

Figure 4.2 – continued

the second to third decade of life and usually in males. Weeks to months later the second eye is involved, although bilateral simultaneous visual loss may occur. Colour vision is severely affected, and perimetry shows either a central or centrocaecal scotoma. Unlike optic neuritis, there is no pain on eye movements and recovery is both exceptional and delayed by months or even years when it occurs. During the acute phase of visual loss circumpapillary telangiectatic microangiopathy may be seen but fluorescein angiography does not show leakage. These fundus appearances are sometimes observed in asymptomatic maternal relatives. However, the absence of these features does not exclude the diagnosis in an individual who loses vision. Eventually optic atrophy with retinal nerve fibre layer defects develops which is

81

particularly obvious in the papillo-macular bundle, often leaving non-glaucomatous disc cupping.

LHON is due to one of a number of point mutations in mitochondrial DNA, most commonly occurring at the 11 778 location with the substitution of adenine for guanine. This mutation has not been found in control subjects. As a consequence, histidine rather than arginine is coded for in subunit 4 of Complex I in the respiratory chain. Why axons of the papillo-macular bundle of the optic nerves should be selectively vulnerable is not understood. About 50% of patients with a clinical picture of LHON and a pathogenic mt-DNA mutation do not have a history of similarly affected relatives, and in these cases the detection of specific mutations is of great diagnostic value. Although LHON is primarily a disease of young males, among those patients in the United Kingdom with the 11 778 mutation, over 25% are female and an overlap syndrome with multiple sclerosis has been described.

Other pathogenic mutations arise at sites 3460 and 14 484. This information carries important prognostic implications. The visual recovery rate may only be 4% in patients with the 11 778 mutation, but up to 37% of those with a defect at site 14 484 may recover. Female involvement in these mutations appears to be rare. The microangiopathy of LHON is less likely to be present in patients with the 14 484 mutation.

Table 4.1   Primary mt-DNA mutations associated with LHON

Primary mutation	Frequency in N. Europe	Recovery rate
11 778	50–60%	2–17%
3 460	15–30%	20–40%
14 484	10%	37–50%

Table 4.2   History of alcohol and tobacco consumption in patients with LHON by mutation

	Tobacco (%)	Alcohol (%)	Both (%)
11 778 ($n = 37$)	49	14	11
3 460 ($n = 7$)	86	50	50
14 484 ($n = 12$)	67	67	58

Source: Riordan-Eva, 1995[9]

In Europe, the 11 778 and 3460 mutations account for at least 90% of families with this disease as defined by a subacute optic neuropathy with a positive maternal family history. Epigenetic factors are also important and tobacco and alcohol have been reported to play a role in the phenotypic expression of the 3460 and 14 484 mutations. This would explain the association between Leber's disease and heavy tobacco consumption, perhaps in nutritionally deficient patients.[9]

An effective treatment for Leber's disease remains to be found: the use of vitamin B12 is unproved and probably ineffective, but it may be valuable to counsel individuals at risk (after first eye involvement, or unaffected maternal relatives) against tobacco and alcohol use and on the benefits of a balanced diet.

Autosomal recessive optic atrophy

Simple

This entity is occasionally noted in the neonate and termed congenital, but more usually is discovered in infancy before the age of three or four years. Severe but stable visual impairment is the rule and associated nystagmus is variable. Disc pallor and retinal arterial attenuation may suggest a retinal dystrophy such as Leber's congenital amaurosis, but the flash electroretinogram is normal.

Complex

The association of infantile recessive optic atrophy, spino-cerebellar degenerations, and cerebellar ataxia is known as Behr's syndrome. There may be an overlap with Charcot–Marie–Tooth disease. Another association is with *D*iabetes *I*nsipidis, *D*iabetes *M*ellitus (*Optic A*trophy) and sensorineural *D*eafness (DIDMOAD, or Wolfram's syndrome).[10] Genetic studies have now established that Wolfram's syndrome is linked to chromosome 4.

Autosomal dominant optic atrophy

The autosomal dominant form of optic atrophy (ADOA) is less severe than the recessive, and is also seen much more frequently. The diagnosis can normally be established by applying the following clinical criteria. There is a dominant mode of inheritance; insidious visual loss between the ages of 4 and 8 years; moderate visual acuity reduction in the range of 6/12 to 6/24 (rarely as poor as 6/60) with possible asymmetry; temporal disc pallor with thinning of the papillo-macular bundle; centrocaecal blindspot enlargement with full peripheral fields to white targets; acquired blue–yellow dyschromatopsia. The clinical course is normally mildly progressive and usually the child can manage at a normal school and take up most occupations. Normally the deficit occurs in isolation, but some cases of associated hearing loss and nystagmus have been reported. Recent genetic linkage studies have assigned the gene for ADOA to chromosome 3 and may allow more accurate diagnosis in mildly affected cases.[11]

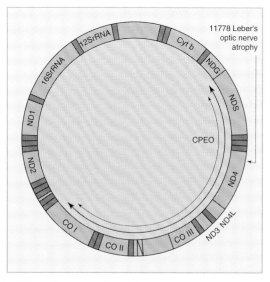

Figure 4.3   Schematic representation of the circular mitochondrial DNA molecule.

4.4   Inflammatory optic neuropathies (optic neuritis)

The differential diagnosis of inflammatory optic neuropathy includes a wide range of immune related, granulomatous, and infective disorders in addition to the common idiopathic form. Most frequently the disc is not swollen, in which case the term retrobulbar neuritis is used.

Typical optic neuritis

Clinical features

In a typical episode of optic neuritis there is an acute or subacute

Table 4.3   Classification of optic neuritis by aetiology

Typical
  idiopathic
  multiple sclerosis
Atypical
  infectious, post-viral and parainfectious
  granulomatous and perineuritis
  autoimmune
  contiguous inflammation of sinuses, meninges or orbit

onset of visual loss progressing over hours or a few days with function reaching its nadir by one week. Unilateral involvement is usual – the less common bilateral disease is a characteristic of the post-viral form, especially in children. Pain on eye movements and mild tenderness of the globe are often present at or shortly before the onset of visual symptoms. Visual loss may range from field and contrast defects with maintained acuity to profound acuity loss with no perception of light. Formal perimetry may show a variety of defects ranging from generalised depression to a central scotoma or altitudinal and nerve fibre layer defects.

Usually vision begins to recover after 2–3 weeks and stabilises by 5–6 weeks. Many patients experience virtually complete restoration of acuity but persistent subtle residual defects of colour vision, contrast sensitivity, depth perception, and cortical evoked potential latency changes are nearly always demonstrable. In some individuals acuity only makes a partial recovery: rarely there is no recovery whatsoever after initial loss. In retrobulbar neuritis, the fundus is by definition normal at the time of onset but subsequently disc pallor may be marked. The final degree of optic atrophy does not correlate closely with the level of visual recovery. In some instances there is also evidence of intraocular inflammation with neuroretinitis and retinal periphlebitis.[12]

In the clinical assessment it is important to establish whether the optic neuritis is isolated or taking place in the context of a systemic illness. The history focuses on other possible CNS lesions by enquiring about paraesthesia, diplopia or unsteadiness; or preceding febrile illness. A typical attack occurs in childhood or adults below the age of 50 years with mild ocular ache and/or pain on eye movements which may reflect the movement of the inflamed nerve within the meninges at the orbital apex. The absence of pain and a failure to follow the typical time course of evolution and recovery of visual loss prompts the careful search for other optic neuropathies – atypical inflammatory lesions, compression by tumours or ischaemia.

Most patients with multiple sclerosis (MS) develop optic neuritis at some stage and 40–70% of patients with clinically isolated optic neuritis go on to develop multiple sclerosis. Subclinical abnormalities of contrast sensitivity and evoked potentials in the fellow eye at the time of acute symptoms imply disseminated white matter lesions in space and time and a diagnosis of MS.[13] Recurrent attacks in the same eye occur in 20–30% of cases but the predictive significance of this for subsequent MS is uncertain. Patients with a clinical picture of neuroretinitis are less likely to develop MS than those with typical optic neuritis: the origins of this variant are more likely to be clearly post-viral.

In our hospital, it is current practice to treat with high dose steroids only those patients with acute optic neuritis who

- have bilateral acute involvement;
- have poor vision in the fellow eye due to some other disease process;
- have a severe visual deficit and severe pain.

Patients with optic neuritis require informed counselling, usually from a neurologist, remembering that MRI abnormalities in the brain at the time of visual symptoms may be associated with increased risk of multiple sclerosis in the future, BUT

1 This cannot be correlated with clinical effects or eventual disease burden.
2 The likelihood of developing multiple sclerosis does not correlate with the likelihood of serious neurological disability.[14]

Devic's disease (neuromyelitis optica)

The association of acute or subacute visual loss due to an optic neuropathy in one or both eyes preceded or followed by transverse or ascending myelitis is known as Devic's disease. In contrast to multiple sclerosis, neuromyelitis optica tends to occur as a single episode without recurrences.

Atypical optic neuritis

- Autoimmune
- Infective
- Granulomatous disease, perineuritis, and "steroid dependent" optic neuropathy
- Paranasal sinus disease and the optic nerve

Systemic lupus erythematosus and systemic vasculitis

The optic neuropathy of systemic lupus erythematosus (SLE) is probably due to small vessel occlusive disease arising either as a consequence of circulating immune complex deposition or to the direct effects of associated anticardiolipin or antiphospholipid antibodies on vascular endothelium and on thrombosis and haemostasis regulation.[15] In Sjögren's syndrome and the vasculitides (polyarteritis nodosa, Churg–Strauss syndrome) primary vessel wall inflammation leads to an ischaemic rather than to a purely inflammatory optic neuropathy. In Behçet's disease, acute disc swelling is more likely to be due to intracranial venous thrombosis and raised intracranial pressure, or an ischaemic process in the optic nerve head.

Post-viral, parainfectious, and infective optic neuropathy

Optic neuritis may follow viral illnesses, in particular chickenpox, rubella, infectious mononucleosis, and mumps, often with full spontaneous recovery. This is the category into which many children with optic neuritis fit, when involvement is frequently bilateral and simultaneous. Postinfective immune mechanisms are suggested by the time course except in herpes zoster ophthalmicus, where the mechanism is more likely to be an associated vasculitis involving the short posterior ciliary vessels.

Other reported causes of "immune" optic neuritis include therapy with interleukin-2, interferon alpha, bee-stings, and the trivalent (MMR) vaccine.

Granulomatous and "steroid dependent" optic neuropathy

In granulomatous optic neuropathy, there is visual loss and disc swelling, either as a result of infiltration of the intraorbital nerve sheath or of the nerve itself.[16] The differential diagnosis includes syphilis, cryptococcus, tuberculosis, sarcoidosis, lymphoma, Wegener's disease, and variants of idiopathic orbital inflammatory disease (pseudotumour). Initial response to steroid treatment may misleadingly mask the underlying diagnosis.

Paranasal sinus disease

Contiguous sinusitis may be important in some optic neuritis patients: the bony wall of the optic canal is often defective medially, leaving the nerve sheath in direct anatomical relationship with the sphenoid sinus. Therefore mucocoeles and pyomucocoeles of the posterior ethmoid and sphenoid sinus may result in optic nerve compression. When orbital cellulitis complicates sinus disease, optic nerve function may fail because of diffuse orbital interstitial pressure rise, intraorbital and subperiosteal abscess formation, as well as posterior ethmoid or sphenoid sinus expansion.[17]

4.5 Ischaemic optic neuropathy

Anterior ischaemic optic neuropathy (AION) due to acute infarction of the optic nerve head is a common cause of visual loss in patients past middle age. Posterior ION is much rarer: the term refers to infarction of the retrobulbar optic nerve without disc swelling.

The blood supply of the optic nerve head is primarily derived from choroidal and posterior ciliary branches of the ophthalmic artery. The posterior ciliary arteries arise independently from the ophthalmic artery and may number from two to four. Usually they form medial and lateral groups, and because they are end arteries a watershed zone is formed between territory perfused by the medial group and territory perfused by the lateral group. When the watershed zone traverses the optic nerve head, this structure is particularly vulnerable to haemodynamic disturbance resulting in infarction and a permanent visual deficit.[18]

AION occurs in two forms: non-arteritic and arteritic, usually due to giant cell arteritis.

Non-arteritic ION

In a typical attack, there is a painless acute onset of loss of acuity and field (usually in an altitudinal pattern) in a patient aged between 50 and 70 years. The onset is acute, first being noticed on awakening, although some patients experience progressive stepwise visual loss over the period of 1–2 weeks. The lack of pain and the age of onset help to distinguish ION from inflammatory optic neuritis. A relative afferent pupil defect indicates that the visual loss is of neuroretinal origin and fundoscopy reveals pallid optic disc swelling which may be sectoral rather than general, often with one or more splinter haemorrhages at the disc margin.

In addition to the risk factors for vascular disease, there is evidence of an anatomical predisposition, as low hypermetropic eyes with small optic discs with low cup–disc ratios ("the disc at risk") are especially vulnerable.[19] The fellow eye is eventually involved in up to 40% of cases.

Arteritic ION (see also Chapters 3 and 9)

In giant cell arteritis (GCA), systemic symptoms of anorexia, malaise, proximal arthralgia, and myalgia (polymyalgia rheumatica), together with headache, scalp tenderness, and jaw claudication, usually precede visual loss. The visual deficit is often severe, with pallid swelling of the entire optic disc and an additional retinal cherry-red spot when ophthalmic artery disease results in a combined posterior ciliary and central retinal artery occlusion.

The management of acute ION consists of:

1 Increase optic nerve head perfusion pressure by measures such as oral or topical carbonic anhydrase inhibitors.
2 High dose corticosteroids and temporal artery biopsy in suspected giant cell arteritis. Normally, this comprises 80 mg prednisolone daily plus 200 mg IV hydrocortisone immediately. When the patient presents with second eye involvement, or the ESR does not fall rapidly after commencing oral steroids, a three day course of pulse IV methyl prednisolone 10 mg/kg is given. A delay of up to 48 hours will not affect the biopsy result after the patient has started corticosteroids. Antiplatelet agents or low dose heparin may also be of value in cases of progressive visual failure.
3 Identification and treatment of systemic vascular risk factors in non-arteritic ION (carotid disease, hypertension, diabetes, prothrombotic states, smoking) to reduce the risk of subsequent stroke.[21]
4 There is no role for optic nerve sheath decompression in ischaemic optic neuropathy, in spite of earlier hopes.[22]

(a)

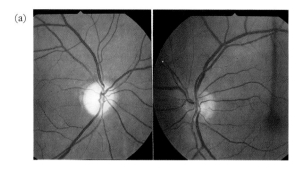

(b)

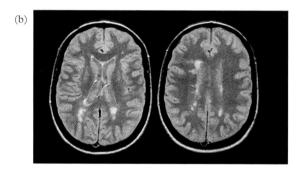

(c)

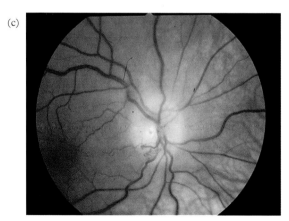

Figure 4.4   continued opposite

(d)

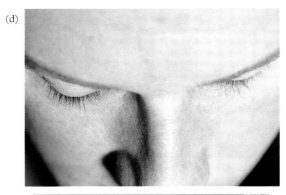

(e)

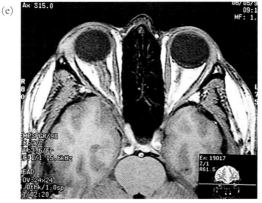

Figure 4.4 (a) Unilateral optic atrophy; (b) periventricular white matter lesions in a proton density axial brain MRI scan of the same patient suggests a diagnosis of multiple sclerosis, but other inflammatory diseases of the CNS are possible; (c) optic disc swelling combined with pallor and a retinochoroidal shunt vessel in a patient with a primary optic nerve sheath meningioma; (d) the same patient viewed from above showing axial proptosis; (e) MRI scan of the orbit of the same patient showing intrinsic optic nerve tumour, shown to be meningioma at excision biopsy.

4.6   Tumours of the optic nerve

Primary optic nerve tumours

Meningiomas
Optic nerve function may be directly impaired by meningiomas arising primarily from the arachnoid cells of the optic nerve sheath, usually in the orbital portions of the nerve. More commonly, however, optic nerve sheath meningiomas arise secondarily from

91

the sphenoid wing, tuberculum sellae or olfactory groove which subsequently invade the optic canal and orbit. Intracranial extension of primary optic nerve sheath meningiomas may also occur. Meningiomas spread along lines of least resistance in the subarachnoid space and are usually encapsulated by intact dura.

Primary optic nerve sheath meningiomas, in common with the same tumour at other sites, most frequently develop in middle aged females. Most tumours are unilateral, but bilateral and multifocal cases exist raising the possibility of an association with central neurofibromatosis (NF2). Clinically there are features of a slowly progressive optic neuropathy with loss of acuity, colour vision, and a central scotoma.

Fundoscopy reveals either simple optic atrophy, or atrophy in association with chronic disc oedema. Retinociliary venous shunt vessels indicating chronic central retinal vein obstruction may appear. Axial proptosis reflecting an intraconal orbital mass is usual in the later stages.

Meningiomas arising from the sphenoid and tuberculum sellae may cause visual failure, either by compression of the intracranial portions of the optic nerve or chiasm, or by intracanalicular and intraorbital extension. In addition, a large inner sphenoid wing meningioma may cause visual loss and anosmia on one side and disc oedema contralaterally (Foster–Kennedy syndrome) as a result of raised intracranial pressure or nerve compression or by a combination of both mechanisms.

Imaging reveals a number of specific features in meningiomas of the orbit. Sphenoid hyperostosis and contrast enhancement on CT are seen in orbital extension of an intracranial mass. In primary optic nerve sheath tumours, tram-line calcification of the orbital optic nerve sheath is a characteristic feature, which will be seen on CT but not on MRI.

The treatment of orbital meningiomas remains controversial. In sphenoid wing tumours which principally have an intracranial component, surgical resection is the treatment of choice.

By contrast, in primary optic nerve sheath meningiomas the surgical approach is not mandatory. No patient is reported to have died from this tumour even after the event of intracranial spread, and the prognosis for vision in the affected eye is very poor, regardless of therapy. There are cases in which, following visual loss from a primary intraorbital lesion, intracranial spread appears to be the next development and radical resection appears to be logical. However, it is important to consider that involvement of the contralateral optic nerve due to spread via the planum sphenoidale has never been clearly documented and surgery is therefore unlikely to influence the likelihood of bilaterality. Bilateral optic nerve sheath meningiomas are thought in fact to arise de novo.[23,24]

Optic and optochiasmal glioma

Primary glial tumours of the anterior visual pathways (optic glioma) are seen in two fundamentally different forms. First, there are benign gliomas of childhood, and secondly there is the rare malignant glioblastoma of adulthood. These are discussed as separate entities, even though they may both present with visual loss and orbital mass effects. Involvement may be of one optic nerve, intraorbital or intracranial, of both optic nerves, of the optic chiasm and of the hypothalamus or thalamus. Malignant optic gliomas of adulthood do not arise from indolent childhood tumours.

Benign optic gliomas of childhood may cause insidious proptosis and visual loss when confined to the orbit. The optic disc may be swollen and/or atrophic and sensory strabismus frequently accompanies visual loss. Progressive proptosis does not necessarily indicate tumour growth, haemorrhage or necrosis. Arachnoid hyperplasia and the extracellular accumulation of periodic acid-schiff (PAS) positive mucopolysaccharide material are characteristic and visual function may fluctuate or even improve spontaneously in some cases. The variable clinical course mitigates in favour of conservative management in most cases.

A careful search for the cutaneous stigmata of NF1 is important. Chiasmal optic gliomas of childhood are commoner than those confined to one optic nerve. Cases present with visual loss, visual field defects and nystagmus. The visual loss is generally bilateral and field analysis may show either central scotomas or temporal hemianopic defects. Nystagmus may be horizontal or rotatory, sometimes with head-nodding mimicking spasmus nutans. A see-saw pattern may also be observed. Features of hypothalamic or thalamic involvement may be present, including the diencephalic syndrome of childhood which includes emaciation and dwarfism in spite of adequate nutrition, skin pallor without anaemia, sleep disturbance and sexual precosity. Hydrocephalus and signs of raised intracranial pressure may develop and leptomeningeal spread has also been reported.

The management of optic glioma has a different emphasis, depending on whether the disease is thought to be purely orbital or intracranial. In intraorbital tumours the role of surgery remains to be fully defined and is generally reserved for palliative treatment in cosmetically unacceptable blind eyes, and the remainder of patients may best be treated conservatively.

In chiasmal glioma, surgical resection is not associated with improved vision or prolonged life. However, surgical intervention may be required for hydrocephalus, decompression of an intraneural cyst or for biopsy when imaging leaves diagnostic doubt. The weight of evidence is now in favour of regarding chiasmal glioma as a benign pilocytic astrocytoma with little tendency to grow. Where growth is clearly documented, radiotherapy may result in tumour shrinkage and visual improvement. However, the benefits must be weighed against the risks of radionecrosis and demyelination at both local and remote sites in an immature brain.

By complete contrast, primary malignant gliomas of the optic nerve have been documented in childhood but generally arise in males aged 40–60 years. Patients present with symptoms and signs that may mimic optic neuritis with rapid monocular visual loss, retrobulbar pain, disc oedema, and transient improvement on corticosteroids, but within several weeks complete blindness and contralateral visual loss ensues. The fundus may show features of central retinal vein or artery occlusion as a result of vascular compression. Radiotherapy and combination chemotherapy may be of some value, but death usually ensues within months and therefore the disease represents the occurrence of a relatively common brain tumour at an uncommon site.[25]

The optic nerve in systemic cancer

Infiltration of the meninges by systemic cancer may sometimes result in painless progressive visual loss due to retrobulbar optic neuropathy. Adenocarcinoma of the breast and lung are the common causes of this syndrome which may be diagnosed by demonstrating meningeal contrast enhancement on MRI together with cytological findings of neoplastic cells in the CSF.[26] Paraneoplastic optic neuropathy has also been described in patients with oat cell carcinoma of the bronchus. In lymphoproliferative disorders the optic nerve may be directly infiltrated, typically with optic disc swelling.[27]

Compressive optic neuropathies

Thyroid ophthalmopathy

Patients with thyroid ophthalmopathy (Graves disease, dys-thyroid eye disease, thyroid eye disease, TED) show signs of orbital congestion, proptosis, and ophthalmoplegia in varying degrees. The extraocular muscles and orbital fat are expanded by inflammatory infiltrate, mucopolysaccharide deposition and, later in the disease process, by fibrotic tissue. The optic nerve may become compressed by swollen muscles and fat at the confined space of the orbital apex. Visual failure most commonly occurs in the inactive, fibrotic phase of the disease, often without conspicuous features of anterior orbital disease (proptosis, lid swelling). However, in some cases, optic nerve compression forms part of the presenting, acute inflammatory phase, in which case chemosis and conjunctival injection, particularly at the sites of insertion of the rectus muscles, are conspicuous. Dyschromatopsia, choroidal folds, and optic disc swelling support the diagnosis, but often fundoscopy is normal. Visual function is best monitored by serial measures of acuity and fields.[28]

Aneurysms and other retrobulbar tumours

The intracranial portion of the optic nerve is intimately related to the major arteries that form the anterior aspect of the basal circle of Willis: the anterior cerebral and anterior communicating arteries, the ophthalmic artery, and the supraclinoid portion of the internal carotid artery itself. Saccular aneurysms may cause a variety of compressive syndromes of the anterior visual pathways, including ipsilateral and contralateral optic neuropathy and/or chiasmal dysfunction.

4.7 Toxic, traumatic, and nutritional optic neuropathies

Slowly progressive bilateral visual loss with central or centrocaecal scotomas and loss of colour vision always suggests the possibility of optic nerve failure due to a toxic cause or nutritional deficiency. A careful family history will exclude heredo-familial disease. In caucasian patients the toxic-nutritional optic neuropathies are usually due to a multifactorial combination of dietary B1 and B2 vitamin complex deficiency, ethanol abuse and high levels of tobacco consumption. Less commonly, malabsorption and vitamin B12 deficiency states produce the same picture.

In other patient populations, additional associations exist. Social dislocation amongst refugee groups in Africa is associated with consumption of uncooked cassava which contains high levels of cyanide. Adequate detoxification mechanisms may be defective when there is an additional B12 deficiency state. HTLV-1 retrovirus infection has been implicated in the syndrome of combined spastic paraparesis and optic neuropathy in African-Americans. A recent epidemic of optic neuropathy in Cuba has been extensively investigated from the point of view of both genetic and environmental factors. Multiple dietary deficiencies have been identified as the probable cause.[29] There is evidence of a possible synergistic effect between dietary deficiencies, mitochondrial DNA mutations and underlying adenosine triphosphate deficiency in the onset of optic neuropathy in some of these patients.[30]

Drug-induced and toxic causes of bilateral optic neuropathy may need careful enquiry to elucidate. Drug-induced disease may be dose dependent (ethambutol, halogenated hydroxyquinolones, and isoniazid), or idiosyncratic (disulfiram, vincristine). Toxins which have been implicated in optic neuropathies include methanol, volatile hydrocarbons, and heavy metals encountered in the course of unprotected occupational exposure or recreational substance abuse.

Traumatic optic neuropathy

Mechanical injury

Mechanical injury to the optic nerve may be direct (penetrating orbitocranial trauma) or indirect. Direct injury is an open wound due to missile injuries or penetrating stab wounds to the orbit. Visual loss is usually instantaneous with impact. Indirect injury is associated with deceleration injuries to the orbital margin or globe which may result in disruption of pial blood supply to the intra-cannicular nerve even in the absence of a fracture.[31]

Radiation injury
See p. 104.

4.8   Applied physiology and clinical features of chiasmal disease

The bitemporal hemianopia is the clinical hallmark of chiasmal lesions, although it is not clear precisely why crossing fibres in the hemidecussation should be selectively vulnerable in both extrinsic and intrinsic disease. In some individuals the intracranial portion of the optic nerves is relatively long and the chiasm is formed in the posterior cistern (post-fixed), with the consequence that expanding sellar lesions may cause optic nerve compression rather than chiasmal compression. Conversely, other individuals may have a pre-fixed chiasm so that mass lesions of the pituitary fossa may impinge on the optic tract. As fibres from the optic nerve enter the chiasm, those serving the nasal and temporal hemiretinas become separated and the anterior nasal projecting fibres loop into the contralateral optic nerve as they cross the midline. Consequently, lesions of the anterior chiasm result in a contralateral temporal hemianopic field defect with an ipsilateral central scotoma. Lesions at the posterior chiasmal notch may selectively involve only dorsal crossing fibres serving central vision resulting in hemianopic scotomata. Macular fibres are present throughout the chiasm and because they serve the central 5 degrees of field and form at least 30% of all the fibres, this has two simple clinical consequences:

1   Chiasmal lesions usually cause defects in central vision (eg acuity or colour tasks) in one or both eyes.
2   Temporal defects respecting the vertical meridian are usually apparent when testing the central visual field if appropriate stimuli are used.

Patients with a bitemporal hemianopia may present with double vision in the presence of normal eye movements. When there are dense temporal field defects, binocular fusion is not supported by overlapping temporal hemifields in the visual cortex. As a result, latent heterophorias may readily break down leading to variable vertical or horizontal diplopia. In other instances there may be difficulties in performing tasks requiring depth perception and judgement. This reflects post-fixational blindness so that when the subject fixates on a near target, objects beyond may project on to both nasal hemiretinas and become invisible. Faulty motion perception may arise as a result of asymmetric optic nerve conduction latencies (Pulfrich phenomenon).

Diplopia may also be paretic: sometimes this is due to a lateral rectus palsy complicating raised intracranial pressure as late presentation occurs with obstructive hydrocephalus. More commonly diplopia reflects parasellar involvement of one or more of the ocular motor nerves, either by compression of the cavernous sinus or direct invasion.

4.9   Visual field testing in suspected chiasmal disease

In the knowledge that the hallmark of chiasmal disease is a bitemporal hemianopia, the clinician may wrongly ascribe every case with bitemporal field loss to chiasmal disease. Bitemporal field defects are also found in

- Massive papilloedema due to blindspot enlargement
- Centrocaecal scotomas
- Tilted, dysplastic optic discs
- Uncorrected refractive errors
- Baggy overhanging upper eyelids
- Bilateral nasal retinal disease (eg sector retinitis pigmentosa).

In practice, these errors are much more likely on confrontation field testing than on some form of quantitative or semi-quantitative testing when close attention is given to ensuring accurate fixation. In this way it can be determined whether or not the defect respects the vertical meridian and thereby can correctly be attributed to a chiasmal rather than to a more anterior cause. However, automated perimetry may create its own problems, for example fixation is checked automatically by retesting stability of the blindspot and this cannot be done in a subject with dense temporal defects. As a rule, we have found the combination of confrontation testing with red-coloured targets, tangent screen testing to a red target, together with perimetry using the manual Goldmann or the automated Humphrey machines, to be much more reliable than any one technique on its own.[32]

4.10   Neuro-imaging in chiasmal disease

Plain skull radiography is no longer performed in suspected chiasmal disease: a normal study does not rule out compression and an abnormal study must always be followed up with imaging. However, imaging must be used with care: not only are clinicians responsible to other patients for the resources they consume but inappropriate imaging may lead to a false sense of security if adequate views of relevant structures are not demonstrated. An unenhanced transverse CT head scan with one cut across the suprasellar region may be normal, but will not necessarily exclude chiasmal compression. The best way to use the powerful tools of high resolution fine cut CT and MRI is to use clinical examination methods to determine whether the problem is optical, retinal, pregeniculate or retrogeniculate and then apply the best techniques available. CT is preferable to MRI for the demonstration of parasellar calcification in a meningioma, craniopharyngioma or aneurysm, or bony destruction and hyperostosis. MRI is superior in demonstrating the relationship of chiasm to tumour mass, showing intrinsic chiasmal lesions and the relationship with adjacent blood vessels. Magnetic resonance angiography (MRA) is likely to replace x-ray angiography in the preoperative distinction between aneurysm and tumour.

4.11 Extrinsic chiasmal disease: tumours and other mass lesions

Pituitary tumours constitute some 12–15% of clinically symptomatic intracranial neoplasms and it has been estimated that up to 20% of all individuals have asymptomatic adenomas at autopsy.

Classification
Clinical classification
   Functional/non-functional
   Microadenoma/macroadenoma (suprasellar extension or not)
   Pituitary apoplexy

Functional classification
   Adenomas with clinically manifest endocrine overactivity
      Growth hormone (acromegaly and giantism)
      Prolactin (galactorrhoea + amenorrhoea in women)
      ACTH (Cushing's disease and Nelson's syndrome)
      TSH and FSH/LH (both very rare)
      Multiple hormones

Adenomas without clinically manifest overactivity
Null cell (may result in hypopituitarism)
Inactive oncocytoma
Prolactin without galactorrhoea
Hyposecretion syndromes

Clinical diagnosis

Patients may present with visual symptoms as discussed above, or may develop headache and/or symptoms and signs of endocrine hypofunction such as loss of secondary sexual characteristics and impotence in men and secondary amenorrhoea in women. Uncommonly, presentation is by downwards invasion into the sphenoid sinus causing epistaxis and nasal obstruction or CSF rhinorrhoea. In functioning tumours a number of specific syndromes arise as listed above. Nowadays, with the increasing use of endocrine testing in the evaluation of patients with infertility and other problems, a higher proportion of pituitary adenomas present before they cause visual failure. When patients present to the endocrinologist with a functioning tumour it is important to determine whether or not there is suprasellar extension (a macroadenoma) so as to assess the risks of subsequent visual failure even if there is no deficit at presentation. This is best done by imaging because an adenoma must extend a full 10 mm across the normal suprasellar cistern before reaching the chiasm. At present even the best imaging may not clearly discriminate a microadenoma from adjacent healthy anterior pituitary tissue.

Medical therapy

Prolactin and many growth hormone secreting microadenomas respond to bromocriptine and other dopaminergic agonists both in terms of reduced secretion and tumour bulk. This approach can also be used in some functioning macroadenomas even if they present with chiasmal compression. In addition, some patients with macroadenomas and normal peripheral blood hormone levels will have prolactin secreting cell types and may shrink with bromocriptine.[33]

Surgery, radiotherapy, and tumour recurrence

Some 75–95% of patients presenting with visual failure will show improvement in visual acuity and field after surgery regardless of whether transfrontal or trans-sphenoidal techniques are used. This

100

is often almost immediate but may continue for some months. As one would expect, those with longstanding visual loss and optic atrophy are less likely to have a full recovery, but the prognostic significance of these features is hard to gauge in an individual patient. In those who have transfrontal surgery alone, recurrence rates may be between 7 and 35%. If combined with radiotherapy, 5 year recurrences fall to 7–13%. In patients treated by transsphenoidal surgery supplemented by radiotherapy, recurrence rates are less than 10%. The low morbidity of this microsurgical operation means that it can be offered to a wider and wider range of patients, including the elderly, those who cannot tolerate or do not respond to bromocriptine, and those with microadenomas. A transfrontal approach may still be required in large macroadenomas and in those with significant lateral extension.

The optimum method of follow-up to detect recurrence remains to be established. Microadenomas are unlikely to develop into lesions causing visual failure except in pregnancy but reliance on endocrine testing alone is unwise as fluctuations in prolactin or growth hormone levels may be hard to interpret. Repeat imaging is expensive and in the case of CT exposes the patient to excess cumulative doses of radiation. In addition, the functional significance of persistent suprasellar masses can only be determined by formal visual assessment. Vision testing alone is inadequate because of the possibility of tumour recurrence into a previous field defect which will not be detectable by perimetry and because vision may deteriorate without recurrence in instances of chiasmal herniation into an empty sella or anterior visual system radionecrosis. It is our current practice to use a combination of all three methods, emphasising the importance of a multidisciplinary approach to the management of these patients not only in diagnosis but also in follow-up.[34,35]

Pituitary apoplexy

Pituitary apoplexy refers to haemorrhagic infarction and necrosis of a pituitary gland containing an adenoma. In the absence of a tumour, the same event may occur after postpartum haemorrhage (Sheehan's syndrome). The difference is that in patients with a pre-existing tumour, the volume expansion will cause sudden visual loss due to chiasmal compression if it is principally in an upwards direction together with external ophthalmoplegia if in a lateral

101

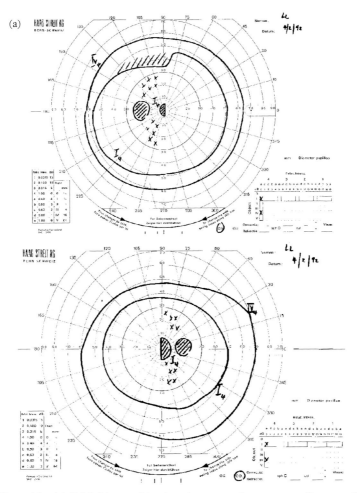

Figure 4.5 (a) Subtle bitemporal hemianopic scotomas due to a suprasellar mass; (b) sagittal MRI brain scan showing a mass expanding from the pituitary fossa to reach and distort the optic chiasm in the same patient; (c) typical Humphrey central threshold fields showing bitemporal hemianopia in a different patient. – continued opposite

direction, whereas in the absence of a tumour the consequences are generally medical from pituitary failure. Where there is ophthalmoplegia, the oculomotor nerve may be especially vulnerable, either because of mechanical compression or because its blood supply depends on meningohypophyseal branches of the internal carotid which may be disrupted. Headache, meningeal

(b)

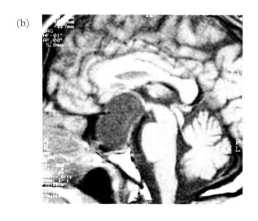

(c)

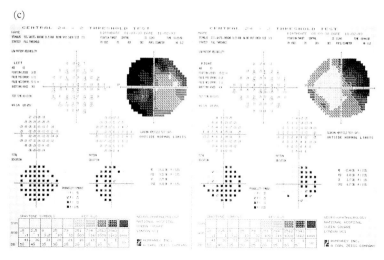

Figure 4.5 – continued

irritation, and drowsiness accompany this event as a result of blood escaping into the subarachnoid space. The diagnosis is made on clinical grounds together with imaging which shows both haemorrhage and features of a pre-existing tumour. Prompt medical measures are required to support pituitary and adrenal function and visual recovery is more likely if early surgical decompression is performed.

Craniopharyngiomas and related lesions (Rathke's cleft cysts and epidermoid cysts)

Craniopharyngiomas, suprasellar epidermoid cysts, and Rathke's cleft cysts are related tumours of embryonic origin arising from vestigial epidermoid remnants of evaginating stomatadeum and Rathke's pouch scattered in the infundibulo-hypophyseal region. Although predominantly arising in the suprasellar region, an intrasellar origin is also possible. In each tumour there is a mixture of solid and cystic elements, typically including fluid filled cysts. In at least 80% of craniopharyngiomas there is dystrophic calcification – a feature of diagnostic importance on CT scanning.

Craniopharyngiomas have a bimodal age distribution of presentation with one peak in childhood and a second in late middle age. They account for some 2–4% of all intracranial tumours, and for over 50% of suprasellar masses in childhood and 20% in adults. In childhood, symptomatic visual loss usually arises quite late and presentation with hypopituitarism and diabetes insipidus or hypothalamic syndromes is typical.

Aneurysms and meningiomas

Giant (ie diameter >25 mm) aneurysms of the supraclinoid carotid artery represent a relatively common and treatable cause of visual loss. They may arise at the origin of the ophthalmic artery (carotid-ophthalmic) or at the bifurcation of the middle cerebral, and tend to expand upwards and forwards to compress the ipsilateral optic nerve and eventually reach the chiasm itself. Parasellar meningiomas expanding upwards may cause similar symptom complexes: surgical "cure" is rarely possible but debulking procedures will reduce morbidity.

4.12   Intrinsic chiasmal lesions

Radionecrosis of the anterior visual pathways

Radionecrosis of the chiasm and intracranial optic nerves is a rare late complication of radiation therapy for sellar, parasellar, and skull base tumours. Visual loss occurs 6 months to 3 years after completion of therapy with a peak incidence between 12 and 18 months. There is no correlation between patient age and the onset of visual loss, which is typically rapid and relentless. Chiasmal, optic tract or unilateral and bilateral optic nerve patterns of loss may be seen. A microvasculopathy and occlusive endarteritis similar to radiation retinopathy is seen following therapy of orbital and nasopharyngeal tumours. The risk is greatest when the total dose is greater than 600 cGy or if fractionated doses are greater than 200 cGy. Hyperbaric oxygen therapy and anticoagulation have both been claimed to improve the final outcome.[36]

Acknowledgement

Figure 4.1(c) is reproduced from Corbett JJ, Savino PJ, Thompson HS *et al. Arch Neurol* 1982;**39**:461–74.

1 Hayreh SS. Pathogenesis of oedema of the optic disc (papilloedema); a preliminary report. *Br J Ophthalmol* 1964;**48**:522–43.
2 Quigley HA, Anderson DR. The histological basis of optic disc pallor. *Am J Ophthalmol* 1977;**83**:709–17.
3 Tso MO. Pathology and pathogenesis of drusen of the optic nerve head. *Ophthalmology* 1981;**88**:1066–80.
4 Wall M, George D. Idiopathic intracranial hypertension: a prospective study of 50 patients. *Brain* 1991;**114**:155–80.
5 Keltner JL. Optic nerve sheath decompression. How does it work? Has its time come? *Arch Ophthalmol* 1988;**106**:1365–9.
6 Acheson JF, Green WT, Sanders MD. Optic nerve sheath decompression for the treatment of visual failure in chronic raised intracranial pressure. *J Neurol Neurosurg Psychiatry* 1994;**57**:1426–9.
7 Lambert SR, Hoyt CS, Narahara MH. Optic nerve hypoplasia. *Surv Ophthalmol* 1987;**32**:1.
8 Hoyt CS, Good CS. Do we really understand the difference between optic nerve hypoplasia and optic atrophy? *Eye* 1992;**6**:201–4.
9 Riordan-Eva P, Sanders MD, Govan GG, Sweeney MG, Da Costa J, Harding AE. The clinical features of Leber's hereditary optic neuropathy defined by the presence of a pathogenic mitochondrial DNA mutation. *Brain* 1995;**118**:319–37.
10 Barrett TG, Bundey SE, Fielder AR, Good PA. Optic atrophy in Wolfram (DIDMOAD) syndrome. *Eye* 1997;**11**:882–8.
11 Johnston RL, Burdon MA, Spalton DJ, Bryant SP, Behnam JT, Seller MJ. Dominant optic atrophy, Kjer-type linkage analysis and clinical features in a large British pedigree. *Arch Ophthalmol* 1997;**115**:100–3.
12 Graham EM, Francis DA, Sanders MD, Rudge P. Ocular inflammatory changes in established multiple sclerosis. *J Neurol Neurosurg Psychiatry* 1989;**52**:1360–3.
13 McDonald WI. The significance of optic neuritis. *Trans Ophthalmol Soc UK* 1983;**103**:230–45.

14 Beck RW, Kupersmith MJ, Cleary PA *et al.* and the Optic Neuritis Study Group. The effects of corticosteroids for acute optic neuritis on the subsequent development of multiple sclerosis. *N Engl J Med* 1993;**329**:1764–9.

15 Cordeiro MJ, Lloyd ME, Spalton DJ, Hughes GRV. Ischaemic optic neuropathy, transverse myelitis and epilepsy in an antiphospholipid positive patient with systemic lupus erythematosus. *J Neurol Neurosurg Psychiatry* 1994;**57**:1142–3.

16 Graham EM, Ellis CJK, Sanders MD, McDonald WI. Optic neuropathy in sarcoidosis. *J Neurol Neurosurg Psychiatry* 1986;**49**: 756–63.

17 Slavin M, Glaser JS. Acute severe irreversible visual loss with sphenoethmoiditis – "Posterior" orbital cellulitis. *Arch Ophthalmol* 1987;**105**:345–8.

18 Hayreh SS. Acute ischaemic optic neuropathy I. Terminology and pathogenesis. *Br J Ophthalmol* 1974;**58**:955–63.

19 Beck RW, Servais GE, Hayreh SS. Acute ischaemic optic neuropathy IX. Cup–disc ratio and its role in the pathogenesis of acute ischaemic optic neuropathy. *Ophthalmology* 1987;**94**:1503–8.

20 Jacobson DM, Slamovits TL. The ESR and its relationship to haematocrit in giant cell arteritis. *Arch Ophthalmol* 1987;**105**:965–7.

21 Hayreh SS, Joos KM, Podhajsky PA, Long CR. Systemic diseases associated with nonarteritic anterior ischaemic optic neuropathy. *Am J Ophthalmol* 1994;**118**:766–80.

22 The Ischemic Optic Neuropathy Decompression Trial Research Group. Optic nerve decompression surgery for nonarteritic anterior ischaemic optic neuropathy (NAION) is not effective and may be harmful. *JAMA* 1995;**273**:625–32.

23 Dutton JJ. Optic nerve sheath meningiomas. *Surv Ophthalmol* 1992; **37**:167–83.

24 Rose GE. Orbital meningiomas: surgery, radiotherapy or hormones? *Br J Ophthalmol* 1993;**77**:313–14.

25 Dutton JJ. Gliomas of the anterior visual pathway. *Surv Ophthalmol* 1994;**38**:427–52.

26 Olson ME, Chernik NL, Posner JB. Infiltration of the leptomeninges by systemic cancer: a clinical and pathologic study. *Arch Neurol* 1974; **30**:122–37.

27 Zaman AG, Graham EM, Sanders MD. Anterior visual system involvement in non-Hodgkin's lymphoma. *Br J Ophthalmol* 1993;**77**: 185–7.

28 Hoh B, Laitt R, Wakeley CJ *et al.* The value of STIR sequence in magnetic resonance imaging of thyroid eye disease. *Eye* 1994;**8**:506–10.

29 Thomas PK, Plant GT, Baxter P, Bates C, Santigo Luis R. An epidemic of optic neuropathy and painful sensory neuropathy in Cuba: clinical aspects. *J Neurol* 1995;**242**:629–38.

30 Rizzo JF. Adenosine triphosphate deficiency: a genre of optic neuropathy. *Neurology* 1995;**45**:11–16.

31 Steinsapir KD, Goldberg RA. Traumatic optic neuropathy. *Surv Ophthalmol* 1994;**38**:478–517.

32 McDonald WI. The symptomatology of tumours of the anterior visual pathways. *Can J Neurol Sci* 1982;**9**:381–9.
33 Moster ML, Savino PJ, Schatz NJ *et al*. Visual function in prolactinoma patients treated with bromocriptine. *Ophthalmology* 1985;**92**:1332–41.
34 Anderson D, Faber P, Marcovitz S *et al*. Pituitary tumors and the ophthalmologist. *Ophthalmology* 1983;**90**:1265–70.
35 Clayton RN, Wass JAH. Pituitary tumours: recommendations for service provision and guidelines for management of patients – commentary. *Eye* 1998;**12**(1):7–8.
36 Zimmerman CF, Schatz NJ, Glaser GS. Magnetic resonance imaging of radiation optic neuropathy. *Am J Ophthalmol* 1990;**110**:389–94.

5: Post-chiasmal disease

JF ACHESON

5.1   Optic tract and lateral geniculate ganglion

Typically, optic tract lesions result in both a non-congruous homonymous hemianopia and in optic atrophy which is most obvious in the contralateral eye. A "bow-tie" (also referred to as band atrophy) pattern is sometimes seen where fibres from the crossing temporal hemifield entering the disc at the 3 o'clock and 9 o'clock positions are lost with preservation of normal disc colour at the upper and lower poles. Because the temporal hemifield served by the nasal hemiretina carries a greater number of ganglion cells which drive the pupillary light reflex than the nasal hemifield, lesions of the optic tract sometimes show a contralateral relative afferent pupil defect.[1,2] This is in distinction to retrogeniculate causes of a homonymous hemianopia where the reflex arc for the pupillary light reflex is typically undisturbed.[3]

Pure optic tract syndromes are uncommon and almost always there are other visual system abnormalities as a result of impairment of adjacent brain stem or chiasm. Tract lesions are typically seen in space occupying suprasellar lesions (pituitary tumours, craniopharyngioma, aneurysms, optochiasmal gliomas) which extend posteriorly, especially when there is a pre-fixed chiasm. Demyelination and vascular occlusion are much less important causes of clinical deficits, although are frequently present at autopsy.

A pure lesion at the lateral geniculate ganglion is even less frequent, and is more often associated with a contralateral hemiparesis from involvement of the adjacent posterior limb of the internal capsule or contralateral hemisensory loss from thalamic involvment. Occlusive vascular disease (hypertension, emboli, vasculitis) of the deep perforating branches of the posterior cerebral (thalamogeniculate and lateral posterior choroidal) artery or anterior choroidal (from the internal carotid) is usually responsible. Horizontal bands of the ganglion may be destroyed resulting in a specific hemianopic wedge field defect (referred to as a geniculate hemianopia), but more often there is a congruous or non-congruous hemianopia. Because the afferent fibres serving the pupillary light reflex exit the tract proximally to the ganglion, a relative afferent pupil defect is not present.[4]

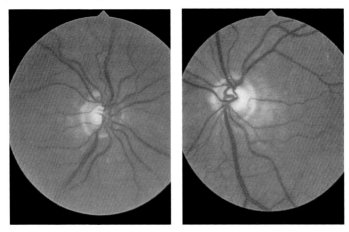

Figure 5.1   Sectoral hemianopia in right lateral geniculate ganglion lesion. (a) Left temporal optic disc pallor; (b) left sectoral hemianopia.

5.2   The visual radiations

Ventral fibres in the geniculo-striate pathway initially pass anteriorly and downwards in the temporal lobe forming Meyer's loop. Lesions in this area usually result in a congruous hemianopia primarily affecting the superior quadrant and with preserved normal visual acuity and pupillary light reflexes. Often there is a wedge shaped extension into the inferior quadrant with a sloping margin. Field defects from lesions in this area arise as a result of intrinsic tumours (gliomas), metastases, and demyelinating plaques more frequently than from vascular occlusion. Temporal lobe surgery for epilepsy will normally spare the geniculo-striate pathways if the resection is confined to the anterior 4–5 cm.

More dorsal fibres pass directly through the parietal lobe and result in a homonymous hemianopia which primarily involves the inferior quadrant, but because the entire geniculo-striate tract passes through the parietal lobe more extensive lesions will cause a total homonymous hemianopia with macular splitting, acuity preservation, and normal pupillary light reflexes. In extensive parietal lesions patients frequently exhibit hemineglect of all sensory modalities together with abnormalities of spatial awareness (apraxia). Ocular motor abnormalities may also arise due to abnormal visual pursuit functions: this is manifested clinically by showing asymmetric responses to the rotating optokinetic drum.

5.3   The primary visual cortex (striate cortex, area V1)

Damage to the visual cortex causes a range of visual disturbances. Classically, attention has focused on various specific patterns of acquired field defect to derive a primary retinotopic map in the striate cortex, which is also known as calcarine cortex, primary visual cortex, Brodmann area 17 and area V1 (see Chapter 1). However, many cortical visual deficits (Table 5.1) cannot simply be understood in terms of field loss, and an awareness of the relationship between the striate and extrastriate cortex is required for an adequate description. Area V1 connects reciprocally with V2, V3, and surrounding areas of visual association cortex. It also connects directly and reciprocally with areas V5 (MT) and at least part of V4. V4 receives both magnocellular (M) and parvocellular (P) inputs, projects ventrally towards the inferotemporal cortex and contains neurones which may contribute to colour and pattern processing. V5 (MT) receives mainly M inputs, projects dorsally towards the occipitoparietal regions and is concerned with processing of motion, attention, and related visuospatial functions.

Field defects in lesions of area V1

Occipital lobe lesions may cause a full congruous homonymous hemianopia or more limited quadrantanopias. If the occipital pole is selectively involved then the macular representation only is affected, causing a hemianopic scotoma.[5] More anterior occipital cortical lesions may produce a monocular defect of the unpaired fibres serving the peripheral temporal hemifield: this is the only exception to the rule that all retrochiasmal lesions result in bilateral field defects. More commonly the reverse syndrome is seen, where the extreme anterior occipital cortex is preserved resulting in a complete homonymous hemianopia except for a temporal crescent of spared vision 60–100 degrees from fixation in one of the otherwise blind hemifields.[6]

Because the occipital pole is served by a dual blood supply deriving from both posterior and middle cerebral artery circulations in some individuals, macular vision may also be preserved in what is otherwise a complete homonymous hemianopia.[7] The precise explanation of "macular sparing" is somewhat controversial (setting aside artifactual cases arising from poor patient fixation which account for the majority), as sparing extends only 10 degrees into the blind hemifield but modern anatomical accounts give at least 60% of the primary visual cortex to this part of the visual field. This extensive portion of cortically magnified visual field in the primary visual cortex probably does not carry a dual blood supply. Earlier theories explaining macular sparing on the basis of bilateral representation of the central vision at both occipital poles have not been substantiated. An overlap of ganglion cell projections from either side of the vertical meridian at the fovea would explain only 1 degree at the most of macular sparing.

Blindsight and stato-kinetic dissociation

"Blindsight", or residual vision in the apparently blind hemifield – a V1 scotoma – continues to generate controversy. Using careful test techniques, a reflex perceptual facility for stimulus presence, location, orientation, direction of movement, and colour can generate appropriate reflex motor responses in spite of deficient conscious awareness. Subcortical pathways from optic tracts to superior colliculi and to the pulvinar of the thalamus have been implicated, as have extrageniculo-striate pathways which project to areas of prestriate cortex (avoiding area V1). Callosal connections accessing the functional capabilities of the intact hemisphere may also play a role.[8]

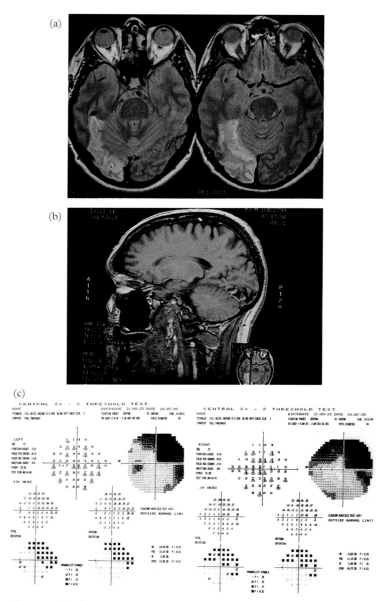

Figure 5.2 Predominantly quadrantic hemianopia in a patient with a stroke affecting the distribution of the inferior calcarine branch of the posterior cerebral artery (note: purely quadrantic defects are more likely to arise from lesions confined to the extrastriate cortex area V2.[10] (a) Axial MRI brain scan; (b) sagittal MRI brain scan; (c) visual field.

A related effect is the Riddoch phenomenon of stato-kinetic dissociation and is demonstrated on Goldmann perimetry, when a stimulus is perceived on movement in the periphery of a homonymous hemianopia despite failure to see colour or static forms.[9]

Bilateral occipital cortex lesions arise quite frequently because the two posterior cerebral arteries are terminal branches of the single basilar artery and therefore basilar occlusions give rise to cortical blindness. A variety of bilateral homonymous lesions ranging from bilateral homonymous hemianopias, bilateral macular sparing homonymous hemianopias (one cause of tunnel vision), quadrantanopias, and scotomas may be seen. When bilateral homonymous hemianopic scotomas arise, a characteristic notch at the vertical meridian betrays the retrochiasmal location of the pathology. The pupillary light reflexes are normal and the visual acuity is usually markedly reduced. Curiously, many patients with cortical blindness may appear to be unaware of their visual loss and use confabulation when asked to perform visual identification tasks. This is known as Anton's syndrome.

Vascular disease accounts for most acquired lesions of the occipital cortex – usually thromboembolism of vertebrobasilar or cardiac origin but all other possible causes of stroke may apply. Because the two occipital lobes together only account for less than 10% of the total cortical volume, tumours are rarely confined to this territory and meningiomas, gliomas, and metastases usually extend into the ipsilateral parietal lobe with associated non-visual symptoms. Bilateral occipital cortex disease also arises in metabolic disease (hypoglycaemia and heavy metal poisoning), neurodegenerative disease (the leukodystrophies, mitochondrial cytopathies) and inflammatory CNS disease (Creutzfeld–Jakob disease, encephalitis, meningitis, demyelination).

5.4 The visual association areas (extrastriate cortex, areas V2–V6)

Areas V2/V3

Lesions affecting human area V1 often extend into underlying white matter, into the prestriate areas (Brodmann 18 and 19), and adjacent parietal and temporal regions. Areas V2/V3 share a common border with V1, which they surround concentrically. Recently, it has been proposed that inferior quadrantic field defects which respect the horizontal as well as the vertical meridian are typical of dorsal V2/V3 lesions.[10]

Areas V4–V6

It is helpful to conceptualise the prestriate pathways, or visual association areas as two separate systems: a ventromesial pathway which occupies the occipital lobe below the calcarine fissure and the adjacent temporal lobe – these areas contain the human homologues of areas V4 in the simian model and IT in the primate model, and a dorsolateral area which is located in the occipital lobe above the calcarine fissures and in the adjacent parietal and temporoparietal-occipital regions – the human homologues of areas V5 and MT. The clinical significance of this is that there may be functional partitioning of the prestriate cortex in such a way that focal lesions may result in selective impairment of aspects of higher visual function.

Ventromesial pathway – cerebral dyschromatopsia and prosopagnosia

Lesions of the ventromesial pathway may result in defects of object recognition, colour vision, and reading. Acquired defects of colour vision are generally the result of lesions of the anterior visual pathways but sometimes cerebral lesions can also cause colour deficits. The human equivalent of area V4 or its white matter connections has been implicated, although the exclusive significance of this territory is disputed. It has been shown that lesions which give rise to loss of colour vision in the contralateral hemifield in humans are located in the ventral occipito-temporal cortex, similar to that activated in normal subjects in positron emission tomography (PET) studies. Pure alexia is frequently associated, as is an impairment of the ability to recognise familiar faces or to learn new faces (prosopagnosia), and typically patients may at the same time have normal acuity, spatial contrast sensitivity, and motion perception. Hemianopic field defects are commonly found, often bilateral inferior quadrantanopias, as a result of damage to the adjacent ventral portions of the optic radiations.[11,12]

Table 5.1   Selected causes of cortical visual disturbances

Vascular
  Posterior cerebral artery occlusion
  Middle cerebral artery occlusion (posterior temporal and parietal branches)
  Watershed zone infarction
  Intracerebral haemorrhage (arteriovenous malformation, hypertension,
    amyloid angiopathy, vasculitis)
  Migraine
Demyelinating disorders
  Multiple sclerosis
  Acute disseminated encephalomyelitis
Degenerative diseases
  Alzheimer's disease
Infections
  Bacterial or fungal abscess
  Viral encephalitis
  Progressive multifocal leucoencephalopathy
  HIV
  Creutzfeldt–Jakob disease
Tumours
  Primary and metastatic
Trauma
  Coup and contracoup
Drug effects
Epilepsy

Dorsolateral pathway – Balint's syndrome, visual agnosia, and cerebral akinetopsia

A further range of selective visual disabilities have been ascribed to lesions of the dorsolateral pathway. These include the visual agnosias where patients have normal visual acuity but cannot identify objects by sight. In Balint's syndrome there is an inability to accurately reach out and grasp objects within the field of view (optic ataxia), an inability to voluntarily reposition gaze to fix on an object of interest (psychic paralysis of gaze), and an unawareness of objects lying to one side of the object of regard in spite of adequate acuity and field (simultanagnosia). Cases of cerebral motion blindness (akinetopsia) have also been reported.[13–15]

Visual hallucinations and miscellaneous disorders

Visual hallucinations occur when the patient reports seeing an image which is not present to any other observer. They are only

115

Table 5.2   Visual disturbances caused by cortical damage

Disorders of colour processing
    Central achromatopsia
    Colour anomia

Disorders of visuospatial processing (localisation, orientation, attention)
    Reduced static visual acuity or contrast sensitivity
    Balint's syndrome
        Simultanagnosia (visual disorientation)
        Optic ataxia
        Optic apraxia
    Metamorphopsia
    Monocular diplopia or polyopia
    Micropsia and macropsia

Disorders of pattern processing and recognition
    Visual agnosia
    Prosopagnosia
    Pure alexia without agraphia

Disorders of temporal processing
    Central akinetopsia (defective motion perception)
    Reduced dynamic visual acuity
    Palinopsia (visual perseveration)

Disorders of stereopsis
    Astereopsis (static or dynamic)

Disorders of visual imagery
    Visual hallucinations

Source: Rizzo M, Nawrot M. Human visual cortex and its disorders. *Curr Opin Ophthalmol* 1993;4(6):38–47

rarely associated with psychiatric disease, in contrast to auditory hallucinations.

Of special interest is the Charles Bonnet syndrome of well-formed visual hallucinations occurring in the elderly with visual loss – both of ocular and neurological origin. Strictly speaking, these are not hallucinations in the neuropsychiatric sense as the subject's insight and mental state is preserved. The patient experiences in vivid detail scenes of faces or complex objects such as fabric patterns or brickwork which are not recognised from previous experience. These tableaux impose themselves on the normally perceived world, usually for only a few minutes at a time, and seem to be related to visual sensory deprivation.[16]

Palinopsia and cerebral diplopia

Palinopsia or visual perseveration causes the patient to continue to perceive an object after it is no longer in view. Usually palinopsia arises as a part of a generalised occipitoparietal syndrome, but is occasionally seen in isolation. The perseverated images may be perceived only in the blind hemifield of a patient with a homonymous hemianopia. A related phenomenon is cerebral diplopia where the patient experiences either monocular diplopia or polyopia in the absence of any abnormality of ocular motility or the intraocular structures (such as astigmatism or lens opacities).[17] The mechanism remains obscure, but probably relates to lesions of V1.

1 Bell RA, Thompson HS. Relative afferent pupillary defect in optic tract hemianopias. *Am J Ophthalmol* 1978;**85**:538–40.
2 Newman SA, Miller NR. Optic tract syndrome: neuro-ophthalmic considerations. *Arch Ophthalmol* 1983;**101**:1241–50.
3 Cibis GW, Campos EC, Aulhorne E. Pupillary hemiakinesia in suprageniculate lesions. *Arch Ophthalmol* 1975;**93**:1322–7.
4 Gunderson CH, Hoyt WF. Geniculate hemianopia: incongruous homonymous field defects in two patients with partial lesions of the lateral geniculate nucleus. *J Neurol Neurosurg Psychiatry* 1971;**24**:1.
5 Trobe JD, Lorber ML, Schlezinger NS. Isolated homonymous hemianopias: a review of 104 cases. *Arch Ophthalmol* 1973;**89**:377–81.
6 Benton S, Levy I, Swash M. Vision in the temporal crescent in occipital infarction. *Brain* 1980;**103**:83–97.
7 Smith CG, Richardson WFG. The course and distribution of the arteries supplying the visual (striate) cortex. *Am J Ophthalmol* 1966; **61**:1391–6.
8 Sanders MD, Warrington EK, Marshall J *et al.* "Blindsight". Vision in a field defect. *Lancet* 1974;**i**:707–8.
9 Safran AB, Glaser JS. Stato-kinetic dissociation in lesions of the anterior visual pathways. *Arch Ophthalmol* 1980;**98**:291–5.
10 Horton JC, Hoyt WF. Quadrantic field defects: a hallmark of lesions in extrastriate (V2/3) cortex. *Brain* 1991;**114**:1703–18.
11 Meadows JC. The anatomical basis of prosopagnosia. *J Neurol Neurosurg Psychiatry* 1974;**37**:489–501.
12 Meadows JC. Disturbed perception of colours associated with localised cerebral lesions. *Brain* 1974;**97**:615–32.
13 Plant GT, Laxter KD, Barbaro NM *et al.* Impaired visual motion perception in the contralateral hemifield following unilateral posterior cerebral lesions in humans. *Brain* 1993;**116**:1303–35.
14 Rizzo M, Nawrot M, Zihl J. Motion and space perception in cerebral akinetopsia. *Brain* 1995;**118**:1105–27.

15 Dutton GN. Cognitive visual dysfunction. *Br J Ophthalmol* 1994;**78**: 723–6.
16 Brown CG, Murphy RP. Visual symptoms associated with choroidal neovascularisation. Photopsias and the Charles Bonnet syndrome. *Arch Ophthalmol* 1992;**110**:1251–6.
17 Bender MB, Feldman M, Sobin AJ. Palinopsia. *Brain* 1968;**91**:321–8.

6: Ocular myopathies, myasthenia gravis, and cranial nerve palsies

LORRAINE CASSIDY

6.1   Ocular myopathies

Degenerative myopathies

Chronic progressive external ophthalmoplegia
Chronic progressive external ophthalmoplegia (CPEO) is characterised clinically by a slowly progressive symmetrical limitation of eye movements. Strabismus and diplopia are rarely seen. Reflecting the infranuclear origin of the ophthalmoplegia, oculocephalic and caloric stimulation do not increase the range of movement. There is usually a symmetrical ptosis and moderate orbicularis oculi weakness in addition. Many patients with CPEO have some degree of retinal pigment epithelial degeneration, ranging from clinically asymptomatic ERG changes, to a mild "salt-and-pepper" retinopathy, and through to a symptomatic field constriction with bone spicules and disc pallor typical of "retinitis pigmentosa".[1] Cardiac conduction defects, cerebellar signs and raised CSF protein may also be present. These additional features have been designated "ophthalmoplegia plus" or Kearnes–Sayre syndrome when the age of onset is under 20 years. Muscle biopsy specimens show the presence of "ragged-red" muscle fibres within

a population of relatively normal fibres on modified Gomori trichrome staining representing degenerate mitochondria. Electron microscopy of apparently normal fibres reveals further abnormal mitochondria. This spectrum of disease is now defined as a mitochondrial cytopathy: in 80–90% of patients with full Kearnes–Sayre syndrome and in 50% with CPEO alone a deletion from mitochondrial DNA can be demonstrated (see Fig. 4.3).[2]

(a)

(b)

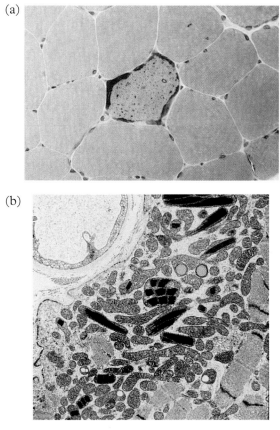

Figure 6.1   (a) A ragged-red muscle fibre with characteristic red peripheral staining in Kearnes–Sayre syndrome (modified Gomori trichrome stain); (b) scanning electron micrograph from same patient showing abnormal mitochondrial inclusions.

Oculopharyngeal dystrophy

This is a hereditary, usually autosomal dominant, muscular dystrophy, in which the bulbar musculature is conspicuously involved causing troublesome dysphagia in addition to external ophthalmoplegia, ptosis and orbicularis weakness.

Myotonic dystrophy

A further cause of external ophthalmoplegia is myotonic dystrophy. Myotonia is the active contraction of a muscle after voluntary cessation of effort or stimulation and may be apparent in the extraocular movements, but typically in the limbs. Patients may have ptosis and myotonia of lid closure in addition to distal muscle atrophy, frontal balding, and endocrine abnormalities. Visual loss results from cataracts and less commonly from retinal pigment epithelial degeneration. An autosomal dominant pattern of inheritance is found with increasing severity of disease and an earlier age of onset in successive generations.

Inflammatory and other myopathies

A variety of other primary muscle diseases cause limited movements and muscle enlargement on imaging[3] and include:

- Orbital myositis
- Thyroid ophthalmopathy
- Parasitosis (trichinosis, echinococcosis)
- Giant cell arteritis
- Primary and secondary neoplasms
- Carotid–cavernous fistula
- Amyloidosis.

A full discussion appears in standard texts on orbital diseases.[4]

6.2   Myasthenia gravis

Definition

Myasthenia gravis is an antibody mediated post-synaptic disorder of the neuromuscular junction causing fatiguable weakness of voluntary muscles due to impaired synaptic transmission of acetyl choline (ACh) across the neuromuscular junction. It may present in early childhood through to extreme old age.[5,6] Transplacental transmission of maternal autoantibodies can cause a self-limiting neonatal myasthenia syndrome.

Pathogenesis

The number of post-synaptic acetyl choline receptors (AChR) at the neuromuscular junction of skeletal muscle is reduced in association with the presence of a polyclonal humoral IgG response and anti-acetyl choline receptor antibodies. Raised levels of antibodies are found in 85% of patients with generalised disease. In the remaining 15% who are seronegative, humoral factors still appear to underlie the disease as patients still respond to plasma exchange and immunosuppression.

The thymus gland is often abnormal, and thymic hyperplasia (characterised by infiltration of the thymus with lymphocytes, plasma cells, and the formation of germinal centres) is observed in 60% of all myasthenics, particularly in the younger age groups, and thymoma (a well-differentiated thymic carcinoma) occurs in 10%. In addition, 5% have autoimmune thyroid disease (which may give rise to an additional ophthalmopathy).

Clinical features

Affected individuals may develop weakness of extraocular, bulbar, and/or limb musculature, which is exacerbated by repetitive or sustained contraction. This weakness may be transiently improved by rest or anticholinesterase agents. Tendon reflexes and sensation are not affected.

Ocular involvement occurs eventually in over 90% of all myasthenic patients and is the presenting complaint (most commonly diplopia or ptosis) in more than 75%.[7] Some (12–15%) patients present with a limited form of myasthenia (ocular myasthenia) in which the disease remains confined to the extraocular muscles, levator palpebrae superioris, and orbicularis oculi, and the anti-AChR antibody levels are low or absent, whilst in other patients there is progression to generalised disease, often within only one or two years.

The clinical features of ocular myasthenia include levator palpebrae superioris involvement with ptosis and a "lid twitch" sign. Some degree of ptosis is almost invariable, and may change from one eye to the other between examinations. The ptosis can also be accentuated by fatiguing movements in which the patient is required to sustain upgaze for a period of more than 30 seconds: this manoeuvre may also provoke an increased vertical squint due to fatigue of elevators of the globe. In a positive lid twitch, after a saccade is made to the primary position from downgaze, the upper lid elevates excessively, and then either slowly becomes ptotic, or twitches a few times before returning to a fixed position.

The extraocular muscle involvement of ocular myasthenia does not follow any set pattern and can mimic a great range of other ocular motility disorders, especially single ocular motor cranial nerve palsies and internuclear ophthalmoplegia. Nystagmus in the abducting eye of a myasthenic – "pseudo internuclear ophthalmoplegia" – may be seen.

Though uncommon, isolated nystagmus may be seen either unilaterally or bilaterally in patients with myasthenia without ophthalmoplegia. Patients with myasthenia may have hypometric large saccades, and hypermetric small saccades. Weakness of the orbicularis oculi is very commonly seen, as shown by ease of prising apart tightly closed lids. Bell's phenomenon may be diminished or absent.

Occasionally, chronic myasthenia may present as an end stage ocular myopathy with severe ptosis, complete external ophthalmo-plegia, and lagophthalmos. A history of fatiguability is absent, the Tensilon is negative, and the distinction between myasthenia and other myopathies (chronic progressive external ophthalmoplegia) can only be made after demonstrating fatigue on single fibre EMG and positive autoantibody assays.

Investigations

Electromyography (EMG) is widely used to support the diagnosis of myasthenia. In ocular myasthenia positive abnormalities such as increased "jitter" within limb muscle may be absent, and single fibre studies of the orbicularis or even the extraocular muscles may be useful.

Tensilon transiently acts to block the action of the enzyme acetyl cholinesterase, thereby making more acetyl choline available at the neuromuscular junction. A negative result does not rule out the diagnosis in the presence of strongly suggestive symptoms and signs. Ten milligrams of intravenous edrophonium will temporarily reverse the muscular weakness so that diplopia and ptosis may resolve. The changing diplopia and range of extraocular movements can be plotted on a Hess chart, but this refinement is difficult to apply in practice because of the variability of these measurements prior to Tensilon, and also because the test may take longer than the 3 minutes available before the effects of the diagnostic injection wear off. Injection of a bolus of edrophonium may be associated with powerful cholinergic cardiac effects and because of the risk of dysrhythmias a test dose of 1–2 mg together with atropine 0.6 mg are given initially in a setting where full resuscitation facilities are quickly available.

Thoracic imaging using CT and MRI to detect a thymoma is routine, although thymoma does not appear to occur in seronegative disease. However, it is not always possible to differentiate between a thymoma and thymic hyperplasia from the scans, especially in young patients.

General principles of treatment

The treatment of myasthenia gravis is the responsibility of the neurologist. Acetylcholinesterase inhibitors are used to improve symptoms and do not prevent progression of disease. Pyridostigmine (Mestinon) and neostigmine (Prostigmin) are two of the more commonly used acetylcholinesterase inhibitors. Inhibition of acetylcholinesterase maximises the availability of ACh to the ACh receptors, hence they can only work when there are receptors present. In very severe myasthenia where there is massive loss of ACh receptors, acetylcholinesterase inhibitors will be of no benefit.

Corticosteroids, and steroid sparing immunosuppressants including cyclosporin and azathioprine, have an important role when symptoms are not adequately controlled by acetylcholinesterase inhibitors, or thymectomy in appropriate cases. Plasmapheresis and intravenous gammaglobulin also have a role in refractory cases. Total thymectomy increases the chances of remission for at least 1–2 years in young seropositive patients, but not when a thymoma is present.

Occasionally, the myasthenia may go into remission and leave the patient with a stable concomitant or paralytic squint which may be amenable to surgical correction.[8] Ptosis props may be used to relieve ptosis but are often poorly tolerated. Ptosis surgery is not recommended, because of the risk of corneal exposure, and the instability of the disease.

Myasthenia-like syndromes

Myasthenic syndromes of fatiguability may arise outside the context of autoimmune disease in paraneoplastic Eaton Lambert syndrome, frequently associated with oat cell carcinoma of the bronchus. There is defective acetylcholine release at the neuromuscular junction. Proximal muscle weakness, which very rarely involves the extraocular and bulbar muscles, is found with absent knee jerks. The muscle weakness seen in these cases tends to improve with muscle contraction.

Drugs including penicillamine, aminoglycosides, vinca alkaloids and corticosteroids may also cause fatiguable muscle weakness. Corticosteroids may also aggravate autoimmune myasthenia gravis and hospital in-patient monitoring is required if this therapy is to be introduced in case the patient requires ventilatory support in the short term.

6.3   Cranial nerve palsies

Abducens nerve palsies

Abducens palsy arising in the brain stem (nuclear and fascicular lesions)

Applied anatomy   The abducens nerve nucleus is situated in the caudal portion of the paramedian pontine tegmentum beneath the floor of the fourth ventricle. Facial nerve fibres loop around the nucleus before exiting in the cerebellopontine angle. The medial longitudinal fasciculus (MLF) passes medially.

There are two populations of cells in the abducens nucleus: the first forms the VIth nerve and passes ventrally to exit at the pontomedullary junction; the second forms internuclear neurones passing in the MLF to the contralateral medial rectus subnucleus in the oculomotor complex. These arrangements explain how a nuclear lesion of the VIth nerve gives rise to both an horizontal gaze palsy and also, frequently, a lower motor neurone facial nerve palsy.

The blood supply of the pons is clinically important in the understanding of the brain stem vascular syndromes. A paramedian/ basal territory is supplied by short circumferential and direct branches of the basilar artery, and a dorsolateral territory supplied by the anterior inferior cerebellar artery, long circumferential arteries, and the superior cerebellar artery.

The abducens nerve has a long intrapontine course of about 10 mm coming into close contact with brain stem structures including the nucleus of the tractus solitarius, the central tegmental

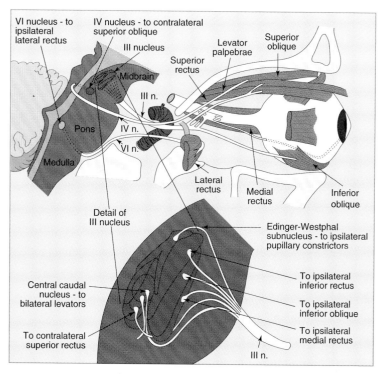

Figure 6.2 Cutaway and sagittal section of brain stem showing organisation of the nucleus of the IIIrd, as well as pathways of the IIIrd, IVth, and VIth nerves from the nuclei to the extraocular muscles.

tract, the spinal tract of the trigeminal nerve, and the superior olivary nucleus. Consequently, lesions of the fascicle are associated with other neurological signs.

Acquired nuclear and fascicular lesions Among the pontine syndromes, *Foville's syndrome* of the anterior inferior cerebellar artery is the commonest whereby a lesion of the pontine tegmentum causes an ipsilateral gaze palsy, lower motor neurone facial palsy, loss of taste in the anterior two-thirds of the tongue, Horner's syndrome, facial analgesia, peripheral deafness or tinnitus and contralateral loss of pain and temperature of the trunk and limbs. Partial forms are more frequent than the full syndrome.

A lesion in the ventral paramedian pons may damage, in addition to the abducens nerve fascicle, the corticospinal tract and/or the

126

Table 6.1   Aetiology of abducens nerve palsy

A: Nuclear (horizontal gaze palsy)	Congenital and hereditary gaze palsies Infarction Tumour Wernicke–Korsakoff syndrome Histiocytosis X
B: Fascicular	Infarction Demyelination Tumour
C: Subarachnoid space	Aneurysms Subarachnoid haemorrhage Trauma Meningitis Clivus tumour Cerebellopontine angle tumours Trigeminal and abducens nerve tumours
D: Petrous	Infection of petrous tip (Gradinego's syndrome) Inferior petrosal sinus thrombosis Trauma Raised intracranial pressure Post-CSF tap Aneurysm and vascular anomaly
E: Cavernous sinus and superior orbital fissure	Carotid aneurysm or dissection Cavernous sinus thrombosis Carotid–cavernous fistula – direct and indirect Tolosa–Hunt syndrome Herpes zoster
F: Orbit	Neoplasms Inflammatory infiltration
G: Non-localising	Microvascular disease (including diabetes, hypertension and vasculitis) Parainfectious Migraine Drugs and toxins

ventral portion of the facial nerve fascicle resulting in an ipsilateral abducens palsy, and contralateral hemiplegia (*Raymond's syndrome*) or additional facial palsy (*Millard–Gubler syndrome*).

Congenital lesions, including Möbius and Duane's syndrome   Isolated congenital paralysis of abduction is exceedingly rare and much more frequently congenital disorders of the abducens nerve are seen together with additional physical signs in the Möbius syndrome and Duane's syndrome.

Table 6.2   Pontine syndromes involving the abducens nerve classified by vascular territory

Vascular territory (syndrome)	Structures involved	Ipsilateral signs	Contralateral signs
Paramedian/basal territory (Millard–Gubler and Raymond syndromes)	VIth fascicle; VIIth fascicle; pyramidal tract	VIth nerve paralysis; VIIth nerve paralysis	Hemiparesis or hemiplegia
Dorsolateral territory (Foville syndrome)	VIth prenuclear fibres/nucleus/ fascicle; VIIth nucleus and fascicle; spinal root of Vth/ spinothalamic tract	Horizontal gaze palsy; VIIth nerve paralysis; hemianaesthesia of face	Hemianaesthesia of limbs

The Möbius syndrome includes facial diplegia and bilateral abducens palsy. Musculoskeletal dysplasias and cleft palate may be associated. Heterogeneous neuropathological findings include hypoplasia or atrophy of cranial nerve nuclei (group I), primary peripheral nerve involvement (group II), brain stem focal necrosis (group III), and myopathies (group IV). Hypoxic or ischaemic insult during pregnancy is implicated in Groups I, II, and III while Group IV patients have fascioscapulohumeral muscular dystrophy. Acquired Möbius syndrome resulting from hypoxic destruction of the internal genu of the facial nerve is described, as are familial patterns of the congenital form.

Duane's syndrome is characterised by limitation or absence of abduction and variable limitation of adduction, together with retraction of the globe and narrowing of the palpebral aperture on attempted adduction of the eye. Duane's syndrome is bilateral in up to 80% of cases. Usually the disorder is sporadic, but familial cases do occur. Numerous ocular, skeletal, and neural abnormalities are associated, notably the Klippel–Fiel anomaly, Goldenhar syndrome, deafness, urinary tract abnormalities, and cardiac defects. These anomalies may be seen singly or in combination throughout certain families and may represent the pleiotrophic effects of the same gene. Autopsy evidence has confirmed that the lateral rectus receives partial or complete innervation from branches of the inferior division of the oculomotor nerve in association with a hypoplastic abducens nucleus and nerve.[9] In one case reported by Miller,[10] the rostral part of the abducens nucleus was preserved, containing the interneurones to the contralateral medial rectus.

The clinical classification of Duane's syndrome is based on clinical findings and electromyography:

- Type I: is by far the commonest, consisting of esotropia with limited abduction caused by lack of lateral rectus firing, mild limitation of adduction with retraction of the globe, and pseudoptosis caused by medial and lateral rectus co-contraction. The medial rectus may be tight.
- Type II: exotropia with limited adduction and retraction on adduction due to co-firing of the medial and lateral recti. The lateral rectus fires in the primary position, accounting for the exotropia, and during abduction with cessation of medial rectus firing. Lateral rectus activity may increase with elevation or depression resulting in A, V and X patterns.
- Type III: a combination of types I and II. There is moderate limitation of abduction and adduction with retraction on adduction due to equal co-innervation of the medial and lateral recti. Both muscles fire in the primary position and on adduction. There is minimal if any firing on abduction. Patients with type III Duane's may be orthophoric, esotopic or exotropic.

Frequently there are vertical deviations of the eye on attempted adduction, thought to be the result of the globe slipping around the tight leash of contracted horizontal recti: these are referred to as upshoots and downshoots.

In contrast to patients with acquired lateral rectus palsy, sensory adaptations are common in Duane's syndrome so that the patient usually does not experience diplopia because of suppression when the affected eye moves into the field of action of the relevant muscle. An abnormal head posture is common in order to maximise binocular function. Most patients with Duane's are more or less orthophoric in the primary position without a noticeable head turn, and are best left alone. Surgery is reserved for those patients who have either a noticeable head turn or a noticeable squint. The aim of surgery is to align the eyes in the primary position, and produce a small horizontal area of binocular single vision. The patient must be warned that they will not have normal eye movements after surgery.

Retraction of the globe on attempted lateral eye movements may also be seen following idiopathic orbital inflammatory disease (orbital pseudotumour), dysthyroid eye disease, and following orbital trauma.

Abducens palsy due to peripheral lesions

Applied anatomy The abducens nerve emerges from the brain stem ventrally and ascends the anterior face of the pons where it is crossed by the anterior inferior cerebellar artery to pierce the dura 2 cm below the posterior clinoids. The abducens nerve traverses or passes above the inferior petrosal sinus and runs beneath the petroclinoid ligament to enter the cavernous sinus. Within the cavernous sinus it lies freely, unsupported by the dural wall. At this point some sympathetic fibres are briefly attached before passing onwards to the ophthalmic trigeminal. From the cavernous sinus, the nerve passes through the annular segment of the superior orbital fissure and innervates only the lateral rectus.

Acquired lesions Within the subarachnoid space the abducens nerve may be damaged by meningeal inflammation and infiltration, fusiform basilar aneurysms, transtentorial cerebral herniation from supratentorial space occupying lesions, and raised intracranial pressure due to other causes.

Lesions at the clivus are often bilateral as both abducens nerves are in close proximity at this point – tumours including meningioma, chordoma, and nasopharyngeal carcinoma may be found.

In the cavernous sinus, the abducens nerve is more vulnerable to compressive effects of mass lesions because it is not tethered to the dural wall, in contrast to the trochlear and oculomotor nerves. The aetiology is frequently an intracavernous vascular lesion (aneurysm or carotid–cavernous fistula), but skull base and parasellar tumours may also be responsible.

Bilateral abducens nerve palsies are commonly due to tumours, demyelination, subarachnoid haemorrhage, meningitis, Wernicke's encephalopathy, and raised intracranial pressure. Bilateral abducens palsy must be differentiated from convergence spasm and divergence paresis.

The age of the patient may be a helpful guide to the likely aetiology. *In infants* VIth nerve palsy must be differentiated from

Duane's syndrome and infantile esotropia with cross fixation. In any child with a sudden ocular deviation efforts must be made to exclude a tumour arising in the retina or anterior visual pathways. Abduction weakness in children may be the first sign of a tumour in the posterior fossa. In these cases a coexistent gaze palsy suggests a pontine glioma, while coexistent cerebellar signs usually indicate astrocytoma, ependymoma or medulloblastoma. In adults aged between 16 and 50 years, vasculopathies, trauma, central nervous system (CNS) inflammatory disease including demyelination and tumours are more likely; in the elderly, degenerative vascular disease is a common cause. In most patients, even when initial investigations including imaging and CSF studies are negative, the cause becomes apparent on careful follow-up and repeat imaging.[11]

Management of unrecovered lateral rectus palsy: general principles
   Several measures are available for the relief of diplopia, abnormal head turns, and eccentric fields of binocular single vision.

1   Base-out prisms or an occluder fitted to spectacle lenses are useful in the acute phase.
2   Botulinum toxin injection to the ipsilateral medial rectus muscle in chronic cases.[12]
3   Extraocular muscle surgery including recession of the overacting ipsilateral medial rectus and resection of the paretic lateral rectus, or muscle transposition of the superior and inferior recti to the affected lateral rectus using adjunctive botulinum toxin chemodenervation to the antagonist medial rectus can be very effective in chronic cases.

Trochlear nerve palsies

Clinical features   Trochlear nerve palsy accounts for the majority of cases with acquired vertical strabismus. Most patients complain of vertical and torsional diplopia that is worse looking down. A head tilt away from the side of the lesion with the chin down is usual with a hypertropia of the affected eye. The hypertropia is maximised on tilting the head towards the side of the lesion and minimised on tilting to the other side. Large degrees of torsion (greater than 10 degrees) suggests a bilateral weakness of the superior obliques, as does a V pattern esotropia.[13]

131

Table 6.3   Aetiology of trochlear nerve palsies

A: Nuclear and fascicular	Congenital aplasia Infarction and arteriovenous malformation Trauma Tumour and other mass lesions Demyelination
B: Subarachnoid space	Trauma Meningitis Tumour Raised intracranial pressure Post-CSF tap
C: Cavernous sinus and superior orbital fissure	Carotid aneurysm Tolosa–Hunt syndrome Herpes zoster Tumours
D: Orbit	Trauma Neoplasms and inflammatory infiltration
E: Non-localising	Microvascular disease (including diabetes, hypertension and vasculitis) Idiopathic

The differential diagnosis of trochlear palsy includes supranuclear skew deviation, thyroid ophthalmopathy, and other restrictive ocular myopathies.[14]

Anatomy   The trochlear nucleus lies in the midbrain at the caudal aspect of the oculomotor nuclear complex. The trochlear fascicles pass dorsally, lateral to the aqueduct to exit the midbrain and cross the contralateral IVth nerve in the anterior medullary velum, just caudal to the inferior colliculi. The trochlear nerve is the only cranial nerve to exit the brain stem dorsally. The nerve continues laterally around the midbrain tectum, crosses the superior cerebellar artery, and reaches the free edge of the tentorium, where it enters the dura and runs forward into the cavernous sinus. The trochlear nerve enters the orbit through the superior orbital fissure, but above the annulus formed by the origin of the rectus muscles, and innervates the superior oblique only.

Congenital lesions   Congenital trochlear nerve palsies are relatively common in contrast to those of the oculomotor and abducens nerves. Often, the cause is a developmental anomaly of the superior oblique tendon in the orbit, but cases of congenital aplasia of the trochlear nucleus have been described. Patients who grow up with a superior oblique deficit undergo a number of sensory adaptations including the development of large vertical fusional amplitudes, which may break down in later adulthood giving rise to symptomatic diplopia. Old photographs will reveal a very longstanding characteristic head tilt. The decompensation is apparently precipitated by age or minor injury.

Nuclear and fascicular lesions

It is virtually impossible to distinguish clinically between nuclear and fascicular lesions of the trochlear nerve with the exception of the combination of unilateral trochlear nerve palsy with a contralateral Horner's syndrome indicating dorsolateral midbrain damage to the fascicle together with the central sympathetic pathways. The trochlear nerve is rarely involved (only 3%) in intrinsic brain stem lesions because of its short intrapontine course. Bilateral trochlear nerve palsies in the absence of a history of trauma may indicate a single lesion of the superior medullary velum.

Peripheral lesions

Trauma accounts for at least 50% of cases. This is said to reflect the susceptibility of the trochlear nerves because of their proximity to the tentorial free margin in the posterior fossa – the tectum of the midbrain suffers a contracoup injury against the tentorial notch and the IVth nerves are damaged either as they sweep laterally around the midbrain, or dorsally in the substance of the superior medullary velum. In this situation, bilateral IVth nerve injury is common. Microvascular ischaemic disease is probably the commonest overall cause after trauma.[15,16]

Management of unrecovered trochlear palsy: general principles

1   Prisms may correct a small vertical deviation in the primary position, but will not correct torsion or increasing diplopia in downgaze.
2   With quantitative measurement of vertical deviations, torsional elements, and fusion it is possible to select patients who may be suitable for extraocular muscle surgery. Weakening of the overacting antagonist inferior oblique, or contralateral synergist inferior rectus is usually preferable to attempts to strengthen the superior oblique.

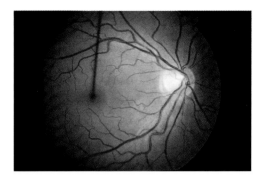

Figure 6.3   Excyclorotation of the right eye in trochlear nerve palsy: note how the optic disc appears to have rotated upwards with respect to the fovea.

Oculomotor nerve palsies

Clinical features   The oculomotor nerve supplies the medial rectus, inferior oblique, inferior rectus, and superior rectus muscles, in addition to the lid levator and the parasympathetic innervation of the pupillary sphincter and ciliary body. A complete IIIrd nerve palsy is easily recognised by the features of ptosis, a fixed dilated pupil and an eye deviated "down and out" with residual function only in abduction (lateral rectus) and intorsion (superior oblique). Incomplete palsies are more common, and careful assessment is essential to avoid confusion with myopathies with selective involvement (myasthenia) or restrictive disease (dysthyroid eye disease and orbital inflammatory disease). Although exceptions are sometimes seen, it is helpful in an emergency to distinguish between "surgical" oculomotor palsies with pupillary involvement and "medical" palsies where the pupil is spared. In the subarachnoid space and cavernous sinus the pupillomotor fibres of the IIIrd nerve lie superficially and dorsally and so are especially vulnerable to a compression from above, such as from a posterior communicating artery aneurysm. By contrast, in microvascular disease the perforating vasa nervorum are occluded primarily, affecting the central fibres and extraocular movements. In cases of acute compression this distinction is less reliable.

134

Table 6.4   Aetiology of oculomotor palsy

A: Nuclear	Congenital aplasia Infarction and arteriovenous malformation Trauma Tumour and other mass lesions
B: Fascicular	Demyelination Haemorrhage Infarction
C: Subarachnoid space (interpeduncular)	Aneurysm – typically posterior communicating artery or basilar artery. Meningitis Microvascular disease – infarction Primary nerve tumours Trauma
D: Tentorial edge	Uncal herniation Raised intracranial pressure Trauma
E: Cavernous sinus and superior orbital fissure	Cavernous sinus thrombosis Carotid aneurysm Tolosa–Hunt syndrome Herpes zoster Tumours Microvascular disease-infarction
F: Orbit	Trauma Neoplasms and inflammatory infiltration
E: Non-localising	Idiopathic Parainfectious Migraine

Nuclear and fascicular lesions: applied neurovascular anatomy

Because vascular occlusion is the commonest cause, a brief overview of applied neurovascular anatomy is appropriate. The upper midbrain and thalamomesencephalic junction are supplied by the posterior subthalamic paramedian branches of the P1 segment of the posterior cerebral artery. In the lower midbrain, three vascular territories can be identified (some accounts give five): the paramedian territory (IIIrd nerve nucleus, part of the medial longitudinal fasciculus (MLF)), supplied by direct twigs coming off the basilar tip, the basal territory (IIIrd nerve fascicular fibres and brachium conjunctivum) supplied by short circumferential branches of the superior cerebellar artery (SCA) and P1, and dorsolateral supplied by the long circumferential branches of the SCA and P1.

Acquired nuclear and fascicular lesions: clinical features Two patterns of ocular motility abnormality are characteristic of lesions of the oculomotor complex:

1 An isolated complete bilateral ptosis. This arises from lesions exclusively affecting the caudal part of the oculomotor nerve complex, where the common cell group for both levator palpebrae superioris muscles lies. Cells for the various extraocular muscles lie rostrally and are not damaged in a purely caudal lesion.
2 A unilateral palsy of the medial rectus, inferior rectus, and inferior oblique together with a contralateral superior rectus palsy. This is seen when one half of the oculomotor complex is damaged: most axons from the subnucleus of the superior rectus decussate to innervate the contralateral muscle.

In Daroff's scheme, a nuclear lesion in oculomotor palsy is certain when there is:

(a) unilateral oculomotor palsy with contralateral superior rectus weakness and bilateral ptosis;
(b) bilateral total oculomotor palsy with spared levator function;

is impossible when there is:

(a) a lateral complete oculomotor palsy with normal contralateral superior rectus function;
(b) unilateral internal ophthalmoplegia;
(c) unilateral ptosis;

and is possible when there is:

(a) bilateral ptosis;
(b) bilateral medial rectus palsy;
(c) bilateral internal ophthalmoplegia;
(d) bilateral total oculomotor palsy.

Nuclear oculomotor palsies are often associated with supranuclear eye movement disorders because of the close relationship to the supranuclear pathways and centres, especially when the cause is infiltrative or neoplastic. Isolated nuclear IIIrd nerve palsies may be seen as a result of selective occlusion of paramedian branches of the basilar artery. Other causes are infection and trauma.[17]

Fascicular lesions of the oculomotor nerve are usually associated with other abnormalities, including contralateral hemiplegia, tremor, and ataxia. There is evidence to suggest the following topographic organisation within the oculomotor nerve fascicle: the most medial fibres are for the pupil, followed by fibres for the inferior rectus, levator, medial rectus, superior rectus, and most laterally, the inferior oblique. Isolated fascicular lesions are caused by infarction, haemorrhage or sometimes demyelination.

Congenital lesions associated with the oculomotor nerve Isolated congenital oculomotor palsy is usually due to perinatal trauma to the peripheral nerve, but absent or incomplete development has been demonstrated in some cases. The pupil is often miotic rather than dilated because of aberrant sphincter innervation. Other misdirection syndromes arise, including:

1 In congenital adduction palsy with synergistic divergence ("the splits") there is a bilateral paralysis of adduction together with bilateral simultaneous abduction on attempted gaze into the field of action of the paretic medial rectus.
2 In the atypical vertical retraction syndrome, co-contraction of superior and inferior rectus muscle results in retraction of the eye into the orbit with narrowing of the palpebral aperture.
3 In cyclic oculomotor paresis with cyclic spasm there is transient oculomotor nerve palsy with ptosis, mydriasis, and ophthalmoplegia, together with involuntary spastic movements in which the eyelid elevates, the pupil constricts, and the eye moves towards the midline, occurring every 2 minutes and lasting for between 10 and 30 seconds. The exact pathogenesis is obscure, but primary (developmental) aberrant regeneration of nuclear and supranuclear fibres is a likely explanation.
4 Jaw-winking synkinesis (trigemino-oculomotor synkinesis, or Marcus Gunn phenomenon) presents as a unilateral ptosis in infancy associated with rhythmic jerking of the upper lid, often as the infant suckles. Some 5% of cases of congenital ptosis are associated with jaw-winking. Two major groups are described: (a) external pterygoid–levator synkinesis with lid elevation when the jaw is moved to the opposite side; (b) internal pterygoid–levator synkinesis with lid elevation on clenching the jaw closed. The first group is the more common.

137

Brain stem syndromes involving the oculomotor nerve These syndromes are only rarely observed in their pure forms and several variations and combinations are possible.

Weber's syndrome, or the syndrome of the cerebral peduncle, is the most frequently observed. It consists of an ipsilateral fascicular oculomotor nerve palsy and a contralateral hemiplegia due to a lesion at the crus cerebri in the ventral part of the mesencephalon. A supranuclear facial palsy may also be present. Partial forms of oculomotor palsy including pupillary sparing are possible, and laterally placed lesions are associated with additional contralateral hypoaesthesia. Infarction of the basal midbrain vascular territory is the usual cause.

Table 6.5   Oculomotor palsies arising in the brain stem classified by vascular territory

Vascular territory (syndrome)	Structures involved	Ipsilateral signs	Contralateral signs
Basal territory (Weber)	IIIrd fascicle, anterior to red nucleus Pyramidal tract	IIIrd nerve paralysis (may be pupil sparing)	Hemiparesis or hemiplegia (hemiparaesthesia)
Paramedian territory (Benedict, Nothnagel, Claude)	IIIrd fascicle, red nucleus, medial lemniscus, substantia nigra	IIIrd nerve paralysis	Extrapyramidal movement disorders (hemianaesthesia)
Dorsolateral territory (Interpeduncular syndrome)	Both IIIrd fascicles Both pyramidal tracts	IIIrd nerve paralysis Hemiplegia/paresis	IIIrd nerve paralysis Hemiplegia/paresis

Benedict's syndrome is characterised by an ipsilateral fascicular oculomotor nerve palsy with a hemiparesis and involuntary movements (hemiballismus or choreoathetosis) contralateral to the lesion due to red nucleus or subthalamic damage. Variants include the Nothnagel syndrome, in which there is ipsilateral cerebellar ataxia, and Claude's syndrome of the red nucleus. Infarction of the paramedian vascular territory is the usual cause.[18]

Acquired peripheral lesions of the oculomotor nerve

Applied anatomy In the interpeduncular space the nerve passes beneath the origin of the posterior cerebral artery and lateral to the posterior communicating artery to run along the free edge of the tentorium and pierce the dura to enter the cavernous sinus lateral to the posterior clinoid. The oculomotor trunk occupies the superior aspect of the cavernous sinus and separates into superior and inferior divisions at about 5 mm before the superior orbital fissure. The inferior branch supplies the medial and inferior recti, the inferior oblique, and the innervation of the ciliary ganglion; the superior branch innervates the superior rectus and levator muscle only.

Clinical features Within the subarachnoid space the oculomotor nerve runs in the subarachnoid space and is vulnerable to meningeal processes such as infection and haemorrhage, and to compression by arterial aneurysm. The commonest site for an aneurysm causing an oculomotor nerve palsy is the internal carotid–posterior communicating artery junction. Usually the pupillomotor fibres are involved in such cases (the "surgical IIIrd nerve palsy"), but especially in the first few days of symptoms the pupil may be spared. Resolution of an oculomotor nerve palsy does not necessarily mean that an aneurysm is excluded, especially if there is a history of facial or orbital pain. Modern neuro-imaging (MR angiography) is normally adequate to exclude an aneurysm without needing to resort to formal angiography. Partial forms of oculomotor palsy may also be due to aneurysm at this site, affecting the superior or inferior division of the nerve, and implying that functionally at least the separation may take place at a more proximal location than the anatomical site before the superior orbital fissure.[19]

The oculomotor nerve may also be compressed against the tentorial edge, petrous ridge, and clivus by the uncus of the temporal lobe during cerebral herniation. Classically the pupillomotor fibres are involved first in this medical emergency. Within the cavernous sinus, the oculomotor nerve may be compressed by infraclinoid carotid aneurysm, when facial pain and trochlear and abducens involvement are common. Pituitary apoplexy and idiopathic inflammatory disease are other causes.

Isolated oculomotor palsy may be due to infarction of the subarachnoid or intracavernous portions, usually in association with diabetes, hypertension or systemic vasculitis. Typically the pupil is spared, reflecting involvement of the perforating vasa nervorum which supply the neurones innervating extraocular muscle fibres.[20] In some cases, nerve infarction arises in the brain

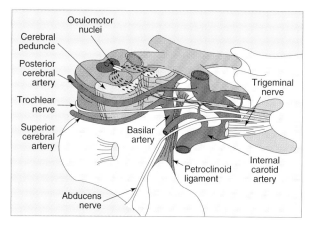

Figure 6.4   Three-dimensional diagram of the course of the right oculomotor nerve in relationship to surrounding structures from the brain stem to the superior orbital fissure.

stem. Trauma may also be responsible – mechanisms include root avulsion at the brain stem origin, or damage at the point of dural perforation or in the supraorbital fissure.

Oculomotor synkinesis   The process whereby, following neuronal damage, regenerating axons may come to innervate structures remote from their original destination is commonly seen following facial nerve injury. Typical examples include intrafacial dyskinesia, paradoxical gustatory sweating, and gustatory tearing. A comparable syndrome arises following oculomotor nerve injury: observed patterns include co-contraction of the levator and medial rectus on attempted adduction or co-contraction of levator and inferior rectus on attempted depression, and pupillary constriction on medial or downward eye movement. Oculomotor synkinesia may be primary or secondary. Primary synkinesia is seen in slowly growing mass lesions of the cavernous sinus, such as a meningioma or infraclinoid aneurysm where there is no prior acute onset of an oculomotor palsy. Secondary synkinesia is seen following incomplete recovery from an oculomotor palsy of acute onset.

Ocular neuromyotonia   Ocular neuromyotonia is a rare disturbance of ocular motility resulting from powerful neuronal discharges from a radiation injured ocular motor nerve causing episodic tonic contraction of the corresponding ocular muscle(s). Most commonly

140

there is a history of radiotherapy for skull base or thalamic tumours. Patients experience intermittent diplopia and may show an intermittent abnormal head posture. The condition has been attributed to anomalous interaxonal connections forming a self-perpetuating reverberating neural circuit.[21]

Ophthalmoplegic migraine and oculomotor palsy in childhood   The syndrome of vomiting, headache, photophobia, and irritability together with pupillary involvement of an oculomotor nerve palsy in children always suggests the possibility of an intracranial aneurysm. However, presentation of berry aneurysms is exceptionally rare in children under 10 years of age, and where a family history of migraine can be elicited and there is rapid resolution of symptoms and signs following a period of sleep, the diagnosis of ophthalmoplegic migraine can be made. The availability of high resolution imaging (usually MRI) means that difficult clinical decisions with regard to angiography are seldom required. In teenagers, aneurysms enter the differential diagnosis as for adults. Other causes of oculomotor palsy in childhood include congenital/developmental anomalies, cranial and orbital trauma, and following viral meningitis. In contrast to abducens palsies, neoplastic disease is a most uncommon cause of a clinically isolated oculomotor palsy.[22]

Management of unrecovered oculomotor palsy: general principles
Some patients are able to allow a complete ptosis to act as an occluder and therefore prevent diplopia. Combinations of horizontal and vertical rectus surgery to both the paretic and non-paretic eye may be helpful, especially in patients with partial palsies.

6.4   Painful and combined ophthalmoplegias

Combined ocular cranial nerve palsies are most commonly unilateral as a result of lesions in the cavernous sinus or superior orbital fissure.[23] In the case of abnormalities located at the superior orbital fissure, proptosis and conjunctival venous congestion may also be seen. Confusion is sometimes caused by the minor degree of proptosis which may accompany loss of tone in multiple extraocular muscles, such as in a complete oculomotor nerve palsy. However, in distinction to true proptosis of orbital disease, resistance to retropulsion of the globe is not seen. Bilateral combined palsies are seen in a diverse range of conditions including postinfectious polyneuropathy (Miller-Fisher variant of Guillain–Barré syndrome), infiltrative brain stem lesions, inflammatory, infective, and neoplastic disease of the basal meninges or cavernous sinus, pituitary apoplexy, and carotid–cavernous fistulas and cavernous sinus thrombosis.

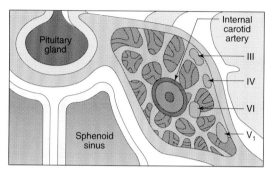

Figure 6.5   Structures within the cavernous sinus showing the position of the oculomotor (IIIrd), trochlear (IVth), abducens (VIth), and ophthalmic (V) nerves within the cavernous sinus.

Painful combined ophthalmoplegias suggest a more specific set of diagnostic possibilities which can be summarised under the headings of inflammatory disease, neoplastic disease, and vascular disease.

Inflammatory disease

Inflammatory disease may be infective or non-infective. In orbital cellulitis a characteristic picture of ophthalmoplegia together with fever, lid swelling, and proptosis complicates local paranasal sinus or metastatic infection. In debilitated patients, orbito-cerebral mucormycosis may present with a similar clinical picture but as the disease progresses ischaemic necrosis of orbital and intraocular structures is a characteristic finding. Commonly, however, the inflammatory process arises apparently without any infective aetiology. The terms "orbital pseudotumour", "idiopathic orbital inflammatory disease" and "Tolosa–Hunt syndrome" are all used in this context. However, it is preferable to describe this group of conditions according to the anatomical location and physical signs encountered: thus orbital myositis, non-infective dacryoadenitis, scleritis, and granulomatous optic perineuritis may each or all be seen in orbital pseudotumour; proptosis, ophthalmoplegia, trigeminal sensory loss, and Horner's syndrome form the superior orbital fissure syndrome; while ophthalmoplegia without proptosis is characteristic of inflammatory disease in the cavernous sinus. Great care is required to exclude the possibility of infective granulomatous disease (tuberculosis), systemic vasculitis (Wegener's granulomatosis) or unsuspected neoplasia (non-Hodgkin's lymphoma and metastases) and a tissue biopsy is often obtained in order to plan definitive treatment in addition to standard imaging.

Neoplastic disease

Although often painless and insidious, primary and metastatic tumours in the cavernous sinus, superior orbital fissure and orbital apex may nevertheless present on occasion with painful ophthalmoplegia. Nasopharyngeal carcinoma, metastatic carcinomas, and invasive squamous cell skin carcinoma are further candidates.

Vascular disease

The constellation of multiple cranial nerve palsies, headache, and variable visual disturbance is strongly suggestive of pituitary apoplexy: by contrast, slowly progressive lateral extrasellar

Table 6.6 Aetiology of multiple ocular motor nerve palsies

A: Brain stem	Encephalitis and AIDS
	Infarction and arteriovenous malformation
	Tumour and other mass lesions
B: Subarachnoid space	Aneurysm
	Meningitis
	Clivus tumours
	Trauma
C: Cavernous sinus and superior orbital fissure	Cavernous sinus thrombosis
	Carotid aneurysm
	Tolosa–Hunt syndrome
	Herpes zoster
	Tumours
	Microvascular disease – infarction
D: Non-localising	Parainfectious (Guillain–Barré and Miller–Fisher syndromes)
E: Orbit	Trauma
	Neoplasms and inflammatory infiltration

expansion of pituitary tumours into the cavernous sinus may be associated with sparing of the function of the oculomotor nerves until late in the disease process. The other vascular lesion of note in the context of painful ophthalmoplegia is infraclinoid (intracavernous) aneurysm. In this condition there is progressive diplopia with features of single and then combined abducens and oculomotor nerve palsies, Horner's syndrome or combined sympathetic and parasympathetic pupillary paresis, trigeminal dysaesthesia, together with periorbital pain which may be severe. Giant infraclinoid carotid aneurysms are typically found in middle aged to elderly women. Meningiomas may sometimes produce a very similar clinical picture, and high resolution imaging together with angiography may be required to make the distinction.

Acknowledgements

Figures 6.2 and 6.4 are reproduced from Slamovits TL, Burde R. *Neuro-ophthalmology*. St Louis: Mosby, 1994.

1 Mullie MA, Harding AE, Petty RKH *et al*. The retinal manifestations of mitochondrial myopathy. *Arch Ophthalmol* 1985;**103**:1825.
2 Holt IJ, Harding AE, Cooper JM *et al*. Mitochondrial myopathies: clinical and biochemical features of 30 patients with major deletions of muscle mitochondrial DNA. *Ann Neurol* 1989;**26**:699–708.
3 Katz B, Leja S, Melles BB, Press GA. Amyloid ophthalmoplegia. Ophthalmoparesis secondary to primary systemic amyloidosis. *J Clin Neurol Ophthalmol* 1989;**9**:39–42.
4 Linberg JV. Diseases of the orbit. In: Tasman W, Jaeger EA, eds. *Duane's clinical ophthalmology, volume 2*. Lippincott-Raven: Philadelphia, 1996.
5 Kaminski HJ, Maas E, Spiegel P, Ruff RL. Why are eye muscles frequently involved in myasthenia gravis? *Neurology* 1990;**40**:1663–9.
6 Weinberg DA, Lesser RL, Vollmer TL. Ocular myasthenia: a protean disorder. *Surv Ophthalmol* 1994;**39**:169–210.
7 Oosterhuis HJGH. The natural course of myasthenia gravis: a long-term follow-up study. *J Neurol Neurosurg Psychiatry* 1989;**52**:1121.
8 Acheson JF, Elston JS, Lee JP, Fells P. Extraocular muscle surgery in myasthenia gravis. *Br J Ophthalmol* 1991;**75**:232–5.
9 Hoyt WF, Nactigäller H. Anomalies of ocular motor nerves. Neuro-anatomic correlates of paradoxical innervation in Duane's syndrome and related congenital ocular motor disorders. *Am J Ophthalmol* 1965; **60**:443–8.
10 Miller NR, Kiel SM, Green WR, Clark AW. Unilateral Duane's retraction syndrome (type I). *Arch Ophthalmol* 1982;**100**:1468–72.

11 Lee J, Harris S, Cohen J, Cooper K, MacEwen C, Jones S. Results of a prospective randomised trial of botulinum toxin therapy in acute unilateral sixth nerve palsy. *J Paediatr Ophthalmol Strabismus* 1994;**31**: 283–6.

12 Savino PJ, Hilker JK, Casell GH, Schatz NJ. Chronic sixth nerve palsies: are they really harbingers of serious disease? *Arch Ophthalmol* 1982;**100**:1442–5.

13 Richards BW, Jones FR, Younge BR. Causes and prognosis in 4278 cases of paralysis of the oculomotor, trochlear and abducens cranial nerves. *Am J Ophthalmol* 1992;**113**:489–96.

14 Spector RH. Vertical diplopia. *Surv Ophthalmol* 1993;**38**:31–62.

15 Brazis PW. Palsies of the trochlear nerve: diagnosis and localisation: recent concepts. *Mayo Clin Proc* 1993;**68**:501–9.

16 Lee J, Flynn JT. Bilateral superior oblique palsies. *Br J Ophthalmol* 1985;**69**:508.

17 Balkan R, Hoyt CS. Associated neurologic abnormalities in congenital third nerve palsies. *Am J Ophthalmol* 1984;**97**:315.

18 Bogousslavsky J, Maeder P, Regli F, Meuli R. Pure midbrain infarction: clinical syndromes, MRI and etiologic patterns. *Neurology* 1994;**44**: 2032–40.

19 Brazis PW. Localisation of lesions of the oculomotor nerve: recent concepts. *Mayo Clin Proc* 1991;**66**:1029–35.

20 Jacobson DM, McCanna TD, Layde PM. Risk factors for ischaemic ocular motor nerve palsies. *Arch Ophthalmol* 1994;**112**:961–6.

21 Ezra E, Spalton D, Sanders MD *et al.* Ocular neuromyotonia. *Br J Ophthalmol* 1996;**80**:350–5.

22 Kodski SR, Younge BR. Acquired oculomotor, trochlear and abducens cranial nerve palsies in pediatric patients. *Am J Ophthalmol* 1992;**114**: 568–74.

23 Rootman J, Nugent R. The classification and management of acute orbital pseudotumors. *Ophthalmology* 1982;**89**:1040.

7: Central disorders of eye movements

TIM MATHEWS

7.1   Saccades
7.2   Smooth pursuit
7.3   Vestibulo-ocular reflex
7.4   Vergence
7.5   Disorders
7.6   Specific patterns of ocular motor deficit

To enable the reader to comprehend the myriad disorders of eye movements, it is necessary to create an understanding of the basic anatomy and physiology of the ocular motor apparatus. There are four main types of eye movement which fall into two broad categories: fast and slow.

1   **Saccades**: To bring an object of attention into foveal vision – *fast*.
2   **Smooth pursuit**: To allow tracking of an object once acquired by the fovea – *slow*.
3   **Vestibulo-ocular reflex**: To compensate for head and body motion stabilising foveal vision in space – *slow*.
4   **Vergence**: To maintain bifoveal fixation of an object as its distance from the viewer changes – *mainly slow*.

These are the prerequisite mechanisms for an eye movement control system in a foveate forward-looking animal.

The analogy of guns on a destroyer at sea acquiring an enemy plane is often used to illustrate these processes. A saccade is the action of the gun acquiring the target when it is first registered. Smooth pursuit is used to maintain the aircraft as the target of the gun after it has been acquired. The vestibulo-ocular reflex is the righting mechanism of the gun that compensates for movement of the ship on the water. Vergence is the process of ensuring guns firing from different locations both track the target when controlled from a single location. Appreciation of the physiology and anatomy of these mechanisms is essential to the understanding of the pathological processes that may disturb them.

All of these processes must overcome two compelling forces within the orbit which act to resist movement of the eyes. The first of these is viscous drag and the second, elastic recoil. Initial movement of the eye is accomplished by overcoming the viscous drag and maintenance of an eccentric gaze position is achieved by resisting the elastic forces within the orbit. Saccades (and their allied movements: the quick phases of nystagmus and the optokinetic reflex) are the only ballistic movement of the eyes and as such are the only movement in which the viscous force is overcome rapidly. All of the other eye movements are non-ballistic or slow and as such the viscous force of the orbit is overcome gradually.

7.1 Saccades

Physiology

Saccades overcome the orbital viscous force by the rapid generation of force within extraocular muscles (phasic contraction). This is achieved by a **pulse** of increased neural activity (see Figure 7.1). This coherent increase in the neural activity of a large pool of oculomotor neurones is produced by specialised cells called **excitatory burst cells** (EBN). To minimise intrusive eye movements during fixation, these cells are kept under tonic inhibitory control by **pause cells** (also called omnidirectional pause cells). A gap in the firing of these cells allows the coherent firing of burst cells producing the ballistic element of the saccade. To maintain the eccentric position of the eye within the orbit, the elastic recoil of the orbital soft tissues must also be overcome. This is accomplished by a **step** increase in the firing rate of the ocular motor neurones producing a tonic contraction of the extraocular muscles (Figure 7.1). The size of the increase in firing rate (ie the size of the step) is derived directly from the size and duration of the pulse. The mathematical term for this derivation is integration. The process of **neural integration**, deriving a position signal from a velocity signal, is performed within the brain stem.

147

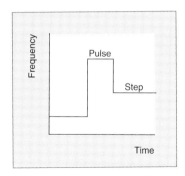

Figure 7.1   Firing frequency of ocular motor neurone during a saccade.

The direct premotor inputs to ocular motor neurones thus come from two sources: the burst cells and the neural integrator. The neural integrator in turn gets its input from the burst cells. As the burst cells are kept under inhibitory control by the pause cells, to generate a saccade another class of cells (long-lead burst neurones) must simultaneously stimulate the appropriate burst cells (direction specific) and interrupt the firing of the pause cells (non-direction specific).

Anatomy

There is an anatomical separation of horizontal (pontine) and vertical (mesencephalic) premotor saccadic centres. Although pause cells for both are located in the nucleus raphe interpositus (between the fascicles of the abducens nerve in the caudal portion of the pontine reticular formation), segregation of the premotor structures is otherwise virtually complete.

Horizontal

Horizontal EBN, which discharge preferentially for ipsilaterally directed saccades, are located in the paramedian pontine reticular formation (PPRF). The output from these cells is directed to two types of neurones that form the abducens nucleus, **motor neurones** that are directed to the ipsilateral lateral rectus and **interneurones** which decussate at the level of the abducens nucleus and ascend in the contralateral median longitudinal fasciculus (**MLF**) to terminate in the contralateral medial rectus subnuclei in the mesencephalon. Neural integration occurs within the medial vestibular nucleus and the adjacent nucleus prepositus hypoglossi.

148

Vertical

Vertical EBN are located in the rostral interstitial nucleus of the MLF (**riMLF**). This nucleus lies at the mesodiencephalic junction dorsal to the red nucleus. Cells on each side discharge for both upward and downward directed saccades but discharge preferentially for torsional movements directed ipsilaterally (ie extortion of the ipsilateral eye and intorsion of the contralateral eye). The output for upward saccades decussates through the posterior commissure whereas the output for downward saccades runs ventrally to the ipsilateral trochlear and inferior rectus subnuclei. The site of the neural integrator for vertical eye movements in man is not yet fully established but it probably resides in the interstitial nucleus of Cajal (**INC**) in the rostral mesencephalon. For both horizontal and vertical eye movements the cerebellum is involved in integrating the output of the burst cells. The output from the cerebellum enters the brain stem at the level of the vestibular nuclei and for vertical movements it then ascends to the INC via the MLF (see below under Internuclear ophthalmoplegia).

Cortical

Cortical control of saccades is also segregated largely between two cortical areas: frontal and parietal. Both have a direct input into the brain stem via the superior colliculus and the frontal cortex additionally relays through the basal ganglia in what appears to be an inhibitory circuit. In subhuman primates and other species there is also a direct input to the PPRF from the frontal cortex, though this has not been clearly established in man. This segregation is functional as well as anatomical. Frontally driven saccades are volitional whereas parietally driven saccades are reflexive.[1]

7.2 Smooth pursuit

Physiology

The purpose of smooth pursuit is to keep an object in clear, foveal, vision as it moves in visual space. This motion may be either predictable or unpredictable. In either case, as smooth pursuit starts it is the movement of the target's image across the

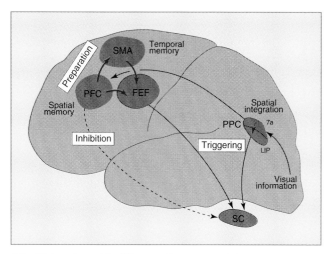

Figure 7.2 Main actions of the different ocular motor cortical areas in saccade initiation. FEF, frontal eye field; LIP, lateral intraparietal area; PFC, prefrontal cortex; PPC, posterior parietal cortex; SC, superior colliculus; SMA, supplementary motor area; 7a, area 7a.

retina which provides the stimulus to the pursuit system. This movement is termed **retinal slip** and the pursuit system uses its speed and direction to produce a corresponding eye movement. To coordinate the movement of the eyes with that of the object, the retinotopic information (the eye's frame of reference) passed to the visual cortex via the magnocellular ganglion cells must be converted into craniotopic information (the head's frame of reference).

The retinal slip stimulus is assessed for direction and speed by direction sensitive cells in the primary visual cortex together with motion sensitive cells in the parieto-occipital junction (area MT in the rhesus monkey or V5 in the macaque). Cells adjacent to MT (area MST in the rhesus monkey) contain information about the position of the eyes and the direction and speed of the target, thus here a craniotopic signal is generated. The primary visual cortex and area MT are responsive only to motion in the contralateral visual hemifield and lesions within them produce a scotoma and a motion detection scotoma respectively in the contralateral hemifield. Area MST is responsive to motion in the whole visual field and a lesion in this area produces a unidirectional defect in pursuit towards the side of the lesion.[2]

In the laboratory we can quantify certain aspects of smooth pursuit: **gain**, **phase**, and **initiation**. Smooth pursuit gain is unity if there is a complete match between target and eye velocity. If eye speed is below target speed, the gain is low and *vice versa*. If the gain is low there will be catch-up saccades. Smooth pursuit phase is a measure of how closely the eye follows the target motion. It is an assessment of the disparity between the position of the eye and the target. If there is no phase shift then the eye and target motion are the same, if there is a negative phase shift then the eye motion lags behind that of the target and *vice versa*. Smooth pursuit initiation is assessed in so-called open-loop experiments in which a stimulus is presented eccentrically and moves with a steady velocity in a given direction (step-ramp).

Anatomy

As there is no need for a ballistic movement, the signal to the brain stem bypasses the burst cells, and feeds into the contralateral cerebellar flocullus, vermis, and uvula, via the ipsilateral dorsolateral pontine nuclei. The dorsolateral pontine nuclei (subadjacent to the abducens nuclei) receive their input from MST and from the frontal eye fields (which in turn receive output from area MT). The output from the cerebellar centres again crosses the midline to terminate in the ipsilateral vestibular nuclei. The output from the vestibular nuclei is then passed to the ocular motor nuclei.

7.3   Vestibulo-ocular reflex

Physiology

The purpose of the vestibulo-ocular reflex (VOR) is to keep the visual scene stable on the retina despite head perturbations. These may occur during head motion alone or as a result of body motion as in locomotion. There are two types of receptors, the three semicircular canals (anterior, posterior, and horizontal; each sensing acceleration in its own plane) and the two otoliths (saccule and utricle; sensing linear motion and head tilt). The construction of the semicircular canals is such that, although they can produce a rapid change in eye position due to direct inputs into the oculomotor circuitry, their output attenuates

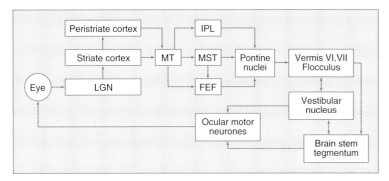

Figure 7.3 Schematic circuit of projections that process visual motion information and generate smooth ocular tracking. Homologous areas for MT and MST of monkey brain are areas 19 and 39 of the human brain, located in the angular gyrus. LGN, lateral geniculate nucleus; MT, middle temporal area; MST, middle superior temporal area; IPL, inferior parietal lobule; FEF, frontal eye field; VI, VII, lobules VI and VII of the vermis in the cerebellum.

with continuing acceleration. As self motion continues another subsystem of vision stabilisation gradually supervenes, and optokinetic nystagmus (OKN) is generated. The output from the vestibular system is already integrated so that a direct head velocity signal is provided. The output from the vestibular nuclei can feed directly into the ocular motor nuclei. There is no cortical routing but their output probably goes through or has a corollary circuit through the cerebellum.

There is a tonic output from each of the sensory areas in the vestibular apparatus which is balanced by an equal output from a corresponding antagonistic receptor during head stability. When the head moves the output from the agonist area increases along with a decrease from the antagonist area. Thus any imbalance from the receptors to the ocular motor nuclei will result in a disturbance of the VOR.

Anatomy

The semicircular canals and otoliths lie within the temporal bone and are connected by the vestibular nerve to the brain stem. The axons from the vestibular apparatus are divided into a superior branch (anterior and lateral canals and utricle) and an inferior branch (superior canal and saccule). These run respectively with the facial nerve and cochlear nerve to the vestibular ganglion at the lateral aspect of the internal auditory meatus. From this location the nerve crosses the cerebellopontine angle to enter the brain stem, between the spinal trigeminal tract and the inferior cerebellar peduncle and terminate in the vestibular nuclear complex. Here the pathway continues directly to the oculomotor nuclei with a corollary output to the gaze holding circuitry for both horizontal (perihypoglossal nuclei) and vertical (interstitial nucleus of Cajal, via the MLF) eye movements.[3]

7.4   Vergence

Physiology

This is the only eye movement system which produces dis-conjugate movements, ie the movements of the two eyes are in different directions; in the case of convergence, towards one another. Vergence is either driven by disparity between the images seen by the two eyes – fusional vergence (vertical, torsional or horizontal) – or is driven by blurring of the visual target – accommodative vergence (horizontal). Usually a combination of the two stimuli leads to vergence movements which enable both foveae to maintain fixation of an object moving in space.

Three classes of vergence premotor neurones have been found:

1   vergence tonic cells which discharge in relation to vergence angle;
2   vergence burst cells which discharge in relation to vergence velocity;
3   vergence burst-tonic cells which discharge in relation to both velocity and angle.

Vergence is one component of the near triad which additionally consists of pupillary miosis and lens accommodation. There is an adaptable relationship between accommodation and accommodative convergence which is assessable clinically and represented as the AC/A ratio.[4]

Anatomy

The majority of vergence movements occur in the horizontal plane, thus for convergence the main excitatory input is to the medial rectus subnuclei and the inhibitory input is to the abducens nuclei. For divergence the reverse is true. The supranuclear premotor pathway for convergence has not yet been established, but it is clear that there is a cortical pathway which probably descends to the mesencephalon directly. The immediate premotor vergence centre is located dorsolaterally to the oculomotor nucleus but the connections both to the oculomotor nucleus and to the abducens nucleus are not formalised. What is clear is that a pathway other than the MLF must carry some if not all of the signal as most MLF lesions do not affect vergence.

7.5   Disorders

Saccades

A lesion in the region of the burst cells will result in a **gaze palsy**, as no pulse will be generated. Lesions to the neural integrator result in **gaze evoked nystagmus**, as it is not possible to overcome the orbital elastic forces (the more severe the lesion the more rapid the slow decay of eye position back to the primary position). Lesions outside the main nuclei (ie the cerebellum) result in **saccadic dysmetria** due to a mismatch between the pulse and step. Lesions in the region of the pause cells will result in **opsoclonus** (back to back saccades) if inhibitory tone is lost, or **slowed saccades** if coherent switching is lost (ie the cells switching off the pause cells do not fire in concert). Failure to generate saccades to command is termed **ocular motor apraxia**: children with developmental delay syndromes may demonstrate abnormal visual behaviour with characteristic head thrusts to refixate the eyes because of a congenital form of this disorder.[5]

Pursuit

A lesion in the motion sensitive cortex (MT) will result in **defective initiation** of smooth pursuit in this area of visual field. A lesion in the adjacent area (MST) will result in a deficit of smooth pursuit in the **contralateral hemifield**. A lesion in the cerebellum will result in low pursuit gain with catch-up saccades – **broken pursuit**.

154

Vestibulo-ocular reflex

A lesion of the semicircular canals or vestibular nerve will give rise to **peripheral vestibular nystagmus** which *worsens* with removal of fixation. This nystagmus has slow phases directed towards the side of the lesion and if the whole nerve is involved it will be a mixture of horizontal and torsional movements. If one semicircular canal or its connections are damaged then the nystagmus will have a plane of motion which is parallel to that of the damaged canal. **Central vestibular nystagmus** is usually either vertical or torsional (or some combination of the two). It is due to lesions of the vestibular nuclei, vestibulo-cerebellum or their onward connections, and *does not worsen* with removal of fixation. **Downbeat nystagmus** may be thought of as a disorder of *posterior* canal connections and **upbeat nystagmus** as a disorder of *anterior* canal projections. In both central and peripheral vestibular lesions **VOR gain** will be disturbed, with a low gain toward the side of the lesion in peripheral disease and a variable effect on gain with central lesions.

A unilateral lesion in the otolith pathway will give rise to an imbalance of graviception with a consequent head tilt, tilt in the subjective visual vertical, and combined torsion and skew deviation of the eyes, the **ocular tilt reaction**.

Vergence

Disorders of the vergence system are usually manifest as **diplopia** or a **squint**. If the defect is acquired the patients usually complain of diplopia or aesthenopic symptoms due to the extra effort to maintain single vision. If the defect is congenital, or acquired prior to visual maturation, the diplopic image may well be suppressed and the defect will be manifest as a squint at a particular viewing distance. Minor head injury and febrile illnesses have been reported to result in symptomatically poor fusional vergence with patients complaining of aesthenopic symptoms or frank diplopia. Thalamic lesions may on occasion cause late-onset concomitant esotropia in childhood.[6]

155

7.6   Specific patterns of ocular motor deficit

Horizontal gaze palsy

In this disorder a lesion has occurred in the final common pathway for horizontal eye movements. The lesion may affect just saccades, in which case it must be located in the PPRF with preservation of the direct smooth pursuit and VOR pathways, or it may affect all eye movements equally, in which case there is a lesion in the VIth nerve nucleus.[7]

Internuclear ophthalmoplegia (INO)

In this disorder a lesion has occurred between the VIth nerve nucleus and the medial rectus subnucleus. The constellation of findings in this condition is due to the amount of neural traffic that takes this route through the brain stem. In addition to slowing of adducting saccades there is often a defect of vertical gaze holding, manifest as upbeating or downbeating nystagmus. There may also be a skew deviation (see below) due to an imbalance of vestibular tone to the INC.[8]

Wall eyed bilateral internuclear ophthalmoplegia (WEBINO)

This is a combination of two INOs and the exotropia, failure of convergence, and vertical gaze instability are a reflection of this. Paralytic pontine exotropia is a closely related condition.[9]

One-and-a-half syndrome

This syndrome comprises a combination of an INO (MLF lesion) and a lesion in the laterally adjacent VIth nerve nucleus or the anteriorly adjacent PPRF. The findings will depend on the exact area of the brain stem affected with a lower motor neurone VIIth lesion often accompanying a VIth nerve nuclear lesion, and a trigeminal tract lesion often accompanying a PPRF lesion.[10]

Vertical gaze palsy

This disorder is usually seen in conjunction with other signs of dorsal mesencephalic disruption. Due to the commissural connections between centres, unilateral lesions may cause unilateral or bilateral defects of upgaze, whereas a bilateral lesion is required to create a bilateral supranuclear downgaze palsy. If vertical VOR or Bell's phenomenon are present then a vertical gaze defect must be supranuclear; however, some patients have been reported with lesions of the supranuclear pathways in whom one or both of these phylogenetically earlier eye movements have been absent.[11]

Parinaud's syndrome or the sylvian aqueduct syndrome

Originally described in association with pineal tuberculomas, this constellation of signs is now recognised as indicating a lesion at the mesodiencephalic junction. The features include a vertical gaze palsy (most usually limited to upgaze) with convergence retraction nystagmus on attempted upgaze, lid retraction (Collier's sign), light–near dissociation, and occasionally spasm of the near reflex. An additional sign to look for is convergence substitution in horizontal movements with slowing of the abducting saccade (so called pseudo-abducens palsy).[12]

Skew deviation

This is defined as a vertical misalignment of the two eyes which cannot be accounted for on the basis of an infranuclear palsy. It may be either concomitant or incomitant and if incomitant may be distinguished from an infranuclear palsy by any associated signs of brain stem dysfunction. A skew deviation represents an imbalance in the vertical vestibular tone between the two sides. A lesion anywhere from the peripheral vestibular apparatus through to the upper midbrain vertical gaze centres may give rise to this clinical sign.[13]

Ocular tilt reaction

In this disorder a skew deviation with concomitant torsion of the eyes (excyclorotation of the hypotropic eye and incyclorotation of the hypertropic eye) is combined with a head tilt towards the hypotropic eye. These lesions have recently been classified into an ascending vestibular type and a descending mesencephalic type.[14]

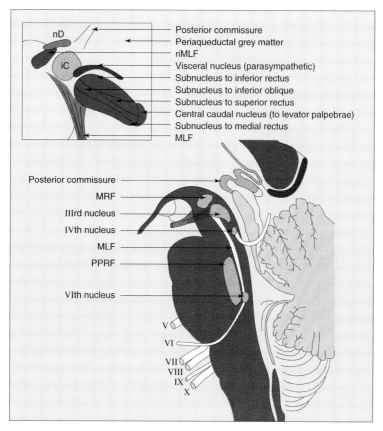

Posterior commissure
Periaqueductal grey matter
riMLF
Visceral nucleus (parasympathetic)
Subnucleus to inferior rectus
Subnucleus to inferior oblique
Subnucleus to superior rectus
Central caudal nucleus (to levator palpebrae)
Subnucleus to medial rectus
MLF

Posterior commissure
MRF
IIIrd nucleus
IVth nucleus
MLF
PPRF
VIth nucleus

V
VI
VII
VIII
IX
X

Figure 7.4   Schematic view of paramedian brain stem structures involved in horizontal and vertical (insert) gaze. Fourth nerve fibres come from the contralateral IVth nerve nucleus, and MLF comes from the contralateral VIth nerve nucleus. (MLF, median longitudinal fasciculus; riMLF, rostral interstitial nucleus of the MLF; PPRF, paramedian pontine reticular formation).

1   Pierrot-Deseilligny C. Cortical control of saccades. *Neuro-Ophthalmol* 1991;**11**:63–75.
2   Leigh RJ. The cortical control of ocular pursuit movements. *Rev Neurol* 1989;**145**:605–12.
3   Leigh RJ, Zee DS. *The neurology of eye movements*, 2nd edn. Philadelphia: F.A. Davis, 1991.
4   Zee DS, Levi L. Neurological aspects of vergence eye movements. *Rev Neurol* 1989;**145**:613–20.
5   Fielder AR, Gresty MA, Dodd KL *et al*. Congenital ocular motor apraxia. *Trans Ophthalmol Soc UK* 1986;**105**:589–96.
6   Williams CS, Hoyt CS. Acute concomitant esotropia in children with brain tumours. *Arch Ophthalmol* 1989;**107**:376–8.

7 Bogousslavsky J, Meienberg O. Eye-movement disorders in brain stem and cerebellar stroke. *Arch Neurol* 1987;**44**:141–8.

8 Sharpe JA, Rosenberg MA, Hoyt WF *et al.* Paralytic pontine exotropia. *Neurology* 1974;**24**:1076–81.

9 Ranalli PJ, Sharpe JA. Vertical vestibulo-ocular reflex, smooth pursuit and eye–head tracking dysfunction in internuclear ophthalmoplegia. *Brain* 1988;**111**:1299–317.

10 Wall M, Wray SH. The one-and-a-half syndrome – a unilateral disorder of the pontine tegmentum: a study of 20 cases and review of the literature. *Neurology* 1983;**33**:971–80.

11 Buttner-Ennever JA, Acheson JF, Buttner U, Graham EM, Leonard TJK, Sanders MD, Ross Russell RW. Ptosis and supranuclear downgaze palsy. *Neurology* 1989;**39**:385–9.

12 Keane JR. The pre-tectal syndrome: 206 patients. *Neurology* 1990;**40**: 684–90.

13 Brandt T, Dietrich M. Different types of skew deviation. *J Neurol Neurosurg Psychiatry* 1991;**54**:549–50.

14 Hedges TR, Hoyt WF. Ocular tilt reaction due to an upper brainstem lesion: paroxysmal skew deviation, torsion, and oscillation of the eyes with head tilt. *Ann Neurol* 1982;**11**:537–40.

8: Nystagmus and other involuntary eye movements

LORRAINE CASSIDY

8.1   Clinical types of nystagmus
8.2   Saccadic abnormalities
8.3   Management of nystagmus and saccadic abnormalities

Nystagmus is an involuntary rhythmic to-and-fro oscillation of the eyes which reflects any disorder of one of several mechanisms that maintain steady gaze. These can be listed as:

1   When the head is still and the eyes are in the primary position, the **visual fixation system** maintains steady gaze.
2   When the eyes are turned to an eccentric position in the orbits, a gaze holding neural network called the **neural integrator** holds steady fixation in this eccentric position.
3   During head rotations, the **vestibular, optokinetic** and **smooth pursuit** systems maintain eyes fixed on a stationary target.

Malfunction of any of these mechanisms results in nystagmus.

Jerk and pendular nystagmus

Jerk nystagmus is characterised by an initial slow phase away from the fixation target, followed by a fast phase back towards the target. The slow phase is mediated by the pursuit system and the fast phase by the saccadic system. The direction of the fast component defines the direction of the nystagmus and the amplitude is normally increased on gaze in the direction of the fast component (Alexander's law).

160

In pendular nystagmus both phases of the oscillation are of equal velocity. The movements may be horizontal, vertical, oblique or rotary. Sometimes fast phases or saccades may be superimposed upon the pendular waveform.

8.1   Clinical types of nystagmus

Nystagmus in normal subjects

Gaze evoked nystagmus in normal subjects

End point nystagmus   Some normal subjects exhibit **end point** or **physiologic** nystagmus. This reflects a short time constant of neural integration, and can be seen with as little as 20 degrees of ocular deviation; however 40 degrees or more of deviation are usually required to induce it. Such nystagmus may be asymmetrical, have a greater amplitude in the abducting eye, and may dampen after several seconds.

Fatigue nystagmus   Results from prolonged (>30 seconds) attempts to maintain extreme lateral gaze in normal subjects.

Optokinetic nystagmus (OKN)
OKN is a jerk nystagmus induced by moving repetitive visual stimuli across the visual field. The fast phase is a saccade and the slow phase a pursuit. Lesions in the occipito-mesencephalic or fronto-mesencephalic pathways result in abnormal OKN responses. Also, the OKN response is difficult to suppress voluntarily and this offers a useful clinical tool (Table 8.1).

Table 8.1   Some clinical applications of testing induced nystagmus with the optokinetic drum

- Pursuit deficits (slow phase) towards the side of the field defect in homonymous hemianopia due to deep parietal lesions
- Asymmetric saccades (fast phase) in internuclear ophthalmoplegia
- Asymmetric pursuit (nasotemporal asymmetry) in congenital esotropia
- Normal nystagmus pattern in functional visual loss

Caloric induced vestibular nystagmus
The patient should be assessed in the supine position with the head 30 degrees from the horizontal (to place the lateral semi-

circular canal in the vertical position). After you have checked that the tympanic membranes are intact, the ears are irrigated with cold and then warm water.

Cold water produces a horizontal jerk nystagmus to the opposite side. Warm water produces a horizontal nystagmus to the same side (mnemonic = COWS – Cold: Opposite; Warm: Same).

When assessing brain stem function in the unconscious patient caloric testing produces no corrective saccade and no nystagmus. Instead, intact vestibular pathways are indicated by a tonic deviation of the eyes to the irrigated side when cold water is used (ie there is only a slow phase and no saccade to the opposite side), and to the opposite side when warm water is used.

Nystagmus in childhood

Congenital nystagmus (CN)

Congenital idiopathic motor nystagmus (CN) can usually be recognised on the basis of a number of characteristic clinical features emphasising the importance of an informed clinical assessment.[1]

Typical CN   In typical CN the age of onset is usually within 3 months of birth and the oscillations have a purely horizontal direction in all positions of gaze. The waveform may be pendular or jerk, or combinations of both. The movements are conjugate, diminish on convergence, and increase on attempted fixation. Frequently, the amplitude varies in different gaze positions and patients often adopt a compensatory head posture to exploit the position with the lowest amplitude (the null point).

CN patients do not experience oscillopsia, but at least 15% have strabismus. "Inverted OKN" or "inverted pursuit" is a feature which seems to be unique to CN: when a patient with CN views a rotating optokinetic drum, the quick phases of their OKN are directed in the same direction as the drum is rotating (ie the opposite to normal).

On formal eye movement recording, a distinctive "CN" waveform is commonly seen, where the velocity increases exponentially to the point of reversal. However, sometimes a pure pendular form may be seen.

162

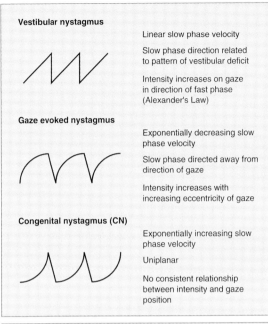

Vestibular nystagmus

Linear slow phase velocity

Slow phase direction related to pattern of vestibular deficit

Intensity increases on gaze in direction of fast phase (Alexander's Law)

Gaze evoked nystagmus

Exponentially decreasing slow phase velocity

Slow phase directed away from direction of gaze

Intensity increases with increasing eccentricity of gaze

Congenital nystagmus (CN)

Exponentially increasing slow phase velocity

Uniplanar

No consistent relationship between intensity and gaze position

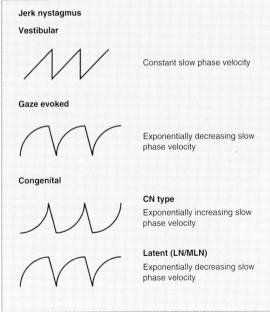

Jerk nystagmus

Vestibular

Constant slow phase velocity

Gaze evoked

Exponentially decreasing slow phase velocity

Congenital

CN type

Exponentially increasing slow phase velocity

Latent (LN/MLN)

Exponentially decreasing slow phase velocity

Figure 8.1   Types of nystagmus.

163

Atypical CN This term is used when the ocular oscillations are not horizontal in all positions of gaze.

A full range of neurophysiological and radiological investigations are required as the child may have eye or brain stem disease, making the diagnosis one of exclusion.

Latent nystagmus (LN) and manifest latent nystagmus (MLN)
Latent nystagmus is a congenital jerk nystagmus which is absent or minimal when both eyes are viewing, and appears or is enhanced when one eye is covered. When one eye is occluded, the fast phase is towards the fixating eye. LN is frequently associated with the congenital esotropia syndrome which frequently also includes dissociated vertical deviation.[2]

LN may become manifest if the patient develops strabismic amblyopia, as the patient is only fixing monocularly. This is termed *manifest latent nystagmus.*

Acquired nystagmus in childhood

Secondary infantile nystagmus Nystagmus may result from any condition which causes reduced vision in early childhood, for example cataract, glaucoma, albinism, retinal dystrophies or aniridia.

Table 8.2   Selected causes of secondary infantile nystagmus

Retina
  Cone dystrophy
  Achromatopsia
  Leber's amaurosis
  Rod monochromacy

Visual pathway
  Optochiasmal glioma
  Craniopharyngioma
  Optic nerve hypoplasia
  Hereditary optic atrophy

Other
  Uncorrected high myopia
  Albinism

As a general rule, if a child loses central acuity before the age of 2 years, nystagmus will always develop. Between the ages of 2 and 6, some will and some will not develop nystagmus. After 6 years nystagmus will not usually occur as a result of visual loss. This is sometimes known as "the 2–4–6 rule".

If there is only partial visual loss, secondary nystagmus may develop before the child has any noticeable difficulty with navigation, and therefore these cases require painstaking clinical examination, often supplemented by electrophysiological testing of the afferent visual system (ERG and VEP) and the ocular motor system (eye movement waveform traces by infrared and video-oculography).

Usually the nystagmus is pendular, and may become jerk on horizontal gaze. Slow wandering conjugate eye movements may be superimposed.[3]

Monocular nystagmus

Uniocular visual loss due to optic glioma may give rise to uniocular nystagmus, but in practice highly asymmetric (atypical) CN is the usual explanation.

Spasmus nutans

This is a term which describes a triad of nystagmus, head-nodding, and abnormal head posture. It characteristically develops in infancy, between 4 and 12 months, and spontaneously resolves before 3 years of age. The nystagmus is characteristically asymmetrical, pendular, with high frequency and low amplitude. This diagnosis can only be made after spontaneous resolution and each child is normally fully investigated at presentation, as for atypical CN and secondary nystagmus.

Nystagmus block syndrome

Refers to a type of congenital nystagmus which is conjugate, horizontal, and associated with an esotropia which has a magnitude inversely proportional to the amplitude of the nystagmus.

The nystagmus is absent or minimal when the fixing eye is in adduction, and becomes more marked when the fixing eye is abducted. Some feel that this may be a form of manifest latent nystagmus.

Acquired horizontal jerk nystagmus

Vestibular nystagmus

Peripheral or central vestibular imbalance results in nystagmus. Disease of the vestibular periphery, ie the labyrinth or the vestibular nerve, results in a unidirectional horizontal nystagmus with the fast phase directed away from the lesion. There is often a torsional component, and this is due to involvement of the posterior semicircular canal. The nystagmus is reduced by visual fixation and is intensified in the dark and on wearing Frenzel goggles (or +20 dioptre lenses which fog out vision). Tinnitus, vertigo, and deafness are commonly present. Saccades and pursuits are normal.

Head movements and posture have a characteristic effect on patients with peripheral vestibular disease:

1   Patients with benign paroxysmal vertigo develop transient nystagmus when lying supine with their head hanging backwards over the top of the examination couch.
2   Transient nystagmus after vigorous head shaking in the horizontal or vertical plane can be induced in patients with a unilateral vestibular lesion.[4]

Gaze evoked or gaze paretic nystagmus

Gaze evoked nystagmus is seen when an attempt is made to maintain an eccentric eye position. The eyes are unable to maintain an eccentric eye position and the orbital elastic tissues cause the eyes to drift back to the primary position. This is followed by a corrective saccade, giving rise to nystagmus. Usually, a supranuclear gaze paresis of smooth pursuit due either to cerebral hemisphere or brain stem lesions is also present.

Gaze evoked nystagmus may be a side effect of many medications including anticonvulsants, sedatives, and alcohol. It can also be caused by lesions of the vestibulocerebellum (flocculonodular node) and within the brain stem.

Combined vestibular and gaze paretic nystagmus

Patients with cerebellar-pontine angle lesions may show both a gaze paretic nystagmus to the side of the lesion as a result of horizontal gaze paresis, together with a faster beating nystagmus in the opposite gaze due to vestibular damage.

Acquired vertical nystagmus

Central vestibular nystagmus

Lesions of the vestibular nucleus or the cerebellar flocculus (vestibulocerebellum) result in a nystagmus which may be bidirectional, purely vertical (up or downbeating), and less commonly torsional or horizontal. Fixation does not reduce the amplitude, and Frenzel goggles or darkness do not intensify the oscillations. Causes include vascular lesions, demyelinating disease, and brain stem tumours.

Downbeat nystagmus

This is a jerk nystagmus with the fast phase downwards. It often presents an exception to Alexander's law by increasing in intensity in lateral gaze.[5] Selected causes are listed in Table 8.3.

Table 8.3   Causes of downbeat nystagmus

Craniocervical junction disease
Arnold–Chiari malformation, Paget's disease, basilar invagination
Cerebellar degeneration
Familial periodic ataxia, paraneoplastic degeneration
Drugs/toxic causes
Lithium, alcohol, B12 deficiency, Mg depletion
Brain stem or cerebellar disease
Infarction, MS, trauma

Upbeat nystagmus

This is a jerk nystagmus with the fast phase beating upwards. When present in the primary position it can be due to a central vestibular lesion. Other causes appear in Table 8.4.

Table 8.4   Causes of upbeat nystagmus

Cerebellar degeneration and inflammation
Multiple sclerosis
Medullary or cerebellar infarction
Posterior fossa tumours
Toxicity
organophosphate poisoning, tobacco, alcohol
Wernicke's encephalopathy

Acquired pendular nystagmus

Acquired pendular nystagmus occurs in three main settings: demyelination, following brain stem stroke, and following monocular visual loss. It may be distinguished from congenital nystagmus, as CN is horizontal, conjugate and tends to convert to jerk in lateral gaze whereas in acquired pendular nystagmus, though occasionally purely horizontal, there are usually vertical and torsional components superimposed. These patients commonly experience severe oscillopsia (the illusion of movement of the seen world as a result of excessive motion of images of stationary objects on the retina) and impairment of visual acuity.[6]

Tremors in other parts of the body such as the palate, head or limbs may coexist. The tremors occur at almost the same frequency as the nystagmus. These patients are said to have ocular myoclonus. In particular, pendular nystagmus can occur in association with palatal myoclonus in patients with multiple sclerosis (MS), and as a delayed consequence of brain stem infarction. This condition is known as oculopalatal myoclonus, and when it occurs after brain stem stroke it is characterised by hypertrophy of the inferior olivary nucleus ("stuffed olive" seen on MRI).

Some special types of nystagmus

See-saw nystagmus

See-saw nystagmus is characterised by the elevation and intorsion of one eye whilst the opposite eye falls and extorts. This occurs in a rapidly alternating sequence. It may be either pendular or jerk. The pendular form is more common and is usually associated with a bitemporal hemianopia resulting from a large suprasellar mass. Other cases are due to lesions within the rostral mesencephalon. Congenital forms may be associated with chiasmal dysplasia.[7]

Periodic alternating nystagmus (PAN)

Acquired PAN is a spontaneous horizontal jerk nystagmus which is present in the primary position of gaze, and changes direction every 90–120 seconds. Usually there is an interval of about 10 seconds before the direction changes in which there may be an up- or downbeating nystagmus, or square wave jerks. A complete cycle takes 4 minutes and may be missed on clinical examination.

Convergence retraction nystagmus

This is characterised by rapid convergence movements of both eyes, which also retract the globes as a result of lesions of the mesencephalon which involve the posterior commissure such as pineal tumours.

Typical associated features include pupillary light–near dissociation, lid retraction, vertical gaze paresis, convergence and accommodation palsy, lid retraction, and skew deviation. Convergence retraction nystagmus is best elicited on attempted voluntary upgaze or with a downwards moving optokinetic drum.

Voluntary nystagmus

These are a series of multiple saccades which can be performed voluntarily by some individuals. They are usually high frequency horizontal conjugate eye movements which appear to be pendular. They may be vertical or even circumrotatory. The individual may have a facial expression of concentration and fluttering lids, and will find these eye movements difficult to sustain for more than a few seconds.

8.2   Saccadic abnormalities

Steady fixation may be disrupted by inappropriate saccades (saccadic intrusions) with different clinical implications than nystagmus.

Square wave jerks and macro-square wave jerks

Square wave jerks are an exaggeration of the normal microsaccadic movements associated with fixation. They consist of a conjugate displacement of 5 degrees of the eyes away from fixation, followed by a refixational saccade after an intersaccadic interval of 200 ms. They are seen in normal healthy subjects and in the elderly. However, if they are more frequent (more than 9 square wave jerks /min in a young person should be considered abnormal), they are referred to as square wave oscillations, and these are seen in cerebellar disease, progressive supranuclear palsy, and multiple sclerosis.

In *macro-square wave jerks* there is a conjugate displacement of the eyes away from fixation by 5 degrees, and after a latency of 80 ms there is a refixation saccade. They occur in bursts and the amplitude is variable, and they are present in the dark. They occur in diseases which disrupt cerebellar outflow such as multiple sclerosis and cerebellar degenerations.

Macrosaccadic oscillations

Here the eyes oscillate conjugately around the fixation (they are a severe form of saccadic hypermetria), with an intersaccadic interval of 200 ms. The oscillations increase and then decrease in amplitude during each episode. They are a result of lesions affecting the midline cerebellum and underlying nuclei. They are not present in darkness.

Ocular dysmetria and ocular flutter

Dysmetria refers to the inability of the saccadic system to bring a target accurately to the fovea. If the target is overshot, a hypermetric saccade has been made. An undershoot is referred to as a hypometric saccade.

Ocular flutter consists of intermittent bursts of binocular to-and-fro saccades with no intersaccadic interval. They occur during straight ahead fixation, and represent an inappropriate firing of burst cells due to a disturbance of the pause cells in the *pontine paramedian reticular formation (PPRF)*. It may be initiated by a blink.

Opsoclonus

This consists of unpredictable continuous conjugate chaotic multidirectional saccades with no intersaccadic interval. They persist during sleep and are indicative of cerebellar disease. It is usually associated with ataxia and may be due to encephalitis or a paraneoplastic process.

Superior oblique myokymia

The syndrome of monocular torsional nystagmus causing intermittent vertical diplopia and oscillopsia is referred to as superior oblique myokymia. Slit lamp examination may be needed to observe these very fine oscillations. The pathophysiology is obscure, but intermittent failure of supranuclear inhibition following a nuclear IVth nerve lesion with subsequent recovery has been postulated. Treatment with carbamazepine or phenytoin may help.

Ocular bobbing and dipping

Typical ocular bobbing consists of rapid conjugate downward jerks followed by a slow upwards drift. The downward jerks may be disconjugate. There is absence of horizontal eye movements.

170

Bobbing usually occurs in comatose patients with extensive intrinsic pontine lesions. A variant form is known as dipping or inverse bobbing and consists of a slow downwards movement, followed by a quick return saccade to the primary position.[8]

8.3 Management of nystagmus and saccadic abnormalities

The aims of treatment are to minimise the sensation of oscillopsia and improve visual acuity.[9]

Pharmacological treatment

Baclofen is effective in the treatment of acquired periodic alternating nystagmus in most cases, but other forms of symptomatic nystagmus are less rewarding to treat. Therapeutic trials with clonazepam, baclofen, scopolamine, valproate, isoniazid, carbamazepine, gabapentin or propranolol may be appropriate. Some patients' visual symptoms improve after alcohol and others deteriorate.[10]

Optical devices

Patients who have a null point at a specific angle may benefit from wearing prisms to place their eyes at the null zone. In some cases of congenital nystagmus a combination of base-out prisms to stimulate convergence together with low myopic lenses to stimulate accommodation and the near triad may improve vision. Contact lenses have been shown to suppress congenital nystagmus in some patients. The mechanism is unclear, but it is thought to be mediated via trigeminal afferents.

Surgery

The null point in congenital nystagmus can be shifted towards the primary position by moving the attachments of the extraocular muscles. This is known as a Kestenbaum or Kestenbaum–Anderson procedure. This involves a recess-resect procedure to rotate the eyes in the direction of the head turn (ie away from the preferred position of gaze or null zone).

Attempts to control oscillopsia by weakening or detaching the rectus muscles or by using botulinum toxin may help in extreme cases, but the results are generally disappointing.[11]

In most patients with acquired nystagmus, treatment of the underlying cause is the only option. For example, foramen magnum decompression for Arnold–Chiari malformation with cerebellar herniation may occasionally improve downbeat nystagmus and prevent the progression of other neurological deficits.

1 Abadi RV, Dickinson CM. Waveform characteristics in congenital nystagmus. *Doc Ophthalmol* 1986;**64**:153–67.
2 Dell'Osso LF, Schmidt D, Daroff RB. Latent, manifest latent and congenital nystagmus. *Arch Ophthalmol* 1979;**97**:1877–85.
3 Weiss A, Biersdorf WR. Visual sensory disorders in congenital nystagmus. *Ophthalmology* 1989;**96**:517–23.
4 Troost BT. Nystagmus: a clinical review. *Rev Neurol (Paris)* 1989;**45**: 417–28.
5 Halmagyi GM, Rudge P, Gresty MA, Sanders MD. Downbeating nystagmus: a review of 62 cases. *Arch Neurol* 1983;**40**:777–84.
6 Gresty MA, Ell JJ, Findley LJ. Acquired pendular nystagmus: its characteristics, localising value and pathophysiology. *J Neurol Neurosurg Psychiatry* 1982;**45**:431–9.
7 Davis, GV, Shock JP. Septo-optic dysplasia associated with see-saw nystagmus. *Arch Ophthalmol* 1975;**93**:137–9.
8 Susac JO, Hoyt WF, Daroff RB, Lawrence W. Clinical spectrum of ocular bobbing. *J Neurol Neurosurg Psychiatry* 1970;**33**:771–5.
9 Leigh RJ, Averbuch-Heller L, Tomsak RL, Remler BR, Yaniglos SS, Dell'Osso LF. Treatment of eye movements that impair vision: strategies based on current concepts of physiology and pharmacology. *Ann Neurol* 1994;**36**:129–41.
10 Averbuch-Heller L, Tusa RJ, Fuhry L, Rottach KG, Ganser GL, Heide W, Buttner U, Leigh RJ. A double-blind controlled study of gabapentin and baclofen as treatment for acquired nystagmus. *Ann Neurol* 1997;**41**:818–25.
11 Tomsak RL, Remler BF, Averbuch-Heller L, Chandran M, Leigh RJ. Unsatisfactory treatment of acquired nystagmus with retrobulbar injection of botulinum toxin. *Am J Ophthalmol* 1995;**119**:489–96.

9: Headache and facial pain

PETER J GOADSBY

The causes and therefore the detailed clinical management of headache and facial pain are myriad. Readers interested in a more detailed clinically orientated analysis of headache are referred to a recent volume[1] and the literature can also satisfy the curiosity of readers wishing to delve deeply into headache from a patho-physiological viewpoint.[2] In this chapter I shall attempt to set out some of the more common, and perhaps not so common but interesting or important, clinical conditions that might result in referral to an ophthalmologist. It is perhaps unfortunate but it has become part of modern folklore that headache is commonly due to ocular disturbances. This provides a constant supply of non-ocular problems with associated headache that may be seen by ophthalmologists. To put headache presentations into context, Table 9.1 outlines the data from a community-based study of headache prevalence which clearly demonstrates that, apart from systemic infections, primary and benign headache dominate the clinical arena.

Clinically, one might divide non-ophthalmological headache and facial pain by the nature of the presentation. Patients are sent for two broad reasons: they have headache or facial pain with some visual disturbance, or there is headache or facial pain and no visual symptoms but the referral was thought to be a good idea. Headache or facial pain as it manifests secondary to

Table 9.1   Common causes of headache

Primary headache		Secondary headache	
Type	Prevalence (%)	Type	Prevalence (%)
Migraine	16	Systemic infection	63
Tension-type	69	Head injury	4
Cluster headache	0.1	Subarachnoid haemorrhage	<1
Idiopathic stabbing	2	Vascular disorders	1
Exertional	1	Brain tumour	0.1

Source: data from Rassmussen[3]

orbital or intraocular disease is covered elsewhere in this volume and will not be further considered.

9.1   General principles of headache and facial pain diagnosis

There are some general rules that assist in diagnosing and therefore correctly managing patients with headache or facial pain syndromes. The many syndromes are laid out in the diagnostic guidelines of the International Headache Society,[4] which serve as a useful reference. There are certain issues which are paramount to establish in the patient presenting with any form of head pain. Perhaps the most important is the length of the history. Patients with a short history require prompt attention and may require quick investigation and management, whereas patients with a longer history require time and patience rather than alacrity. There are some important general features which are perhaps almost too basic but remain at the core of the clinical evaluation. Particular features of importance include associated fever or sudden onset of pain, among others (Table 9.2) and demand attention. With these general rules the specific circumstances can be discussed.

9.2   Headache or facial pain with visual disturbance

Patients with headache or facial pain and associated visual disturbance are frequently referred to ophthalmologists. The visual disturbances which might fall more into the neurological remit can

Table 9.2 Warning signs in head pain

- Sudden onset pain
- Fever
- Marked change in pain character or timing
- Neck stiffness
- Pain associated with higher centre complaints
- Pain associated with neurological disturbance, such as clumsiness or weakness
- Pain associated with local tenderness, such as of the temporal artery

vary from mild recurrent visual blurring to visual impairment which may be intermittent or persistent. Mild visual impairment, such as some blurring of vision, in association with headache brings into consideration a number of problems.

Visual disturbance with headache

It has been considered for some time that convergence weakness or refractive errors may give rise to headache.[5] The headache is described as a dull bilateral band-like headache which can be continuous and can, by definition, be cured by corrective measures. While this syndrome exists it is probably over-emphasised. Comparing patients with no headache and those with frequent headache, as populations, Waters[6] only found hyperphoria with near vision but no other differences in migraine sufferers. It seems likely that mild visual errors might trigger migraine, along with many other triggers, given the correct setting. Furthermore, visual blurring is often seen before or during a migraine attack, so that episodic, perhaps unilateral and throbbing pain with associated features and some visual blurring should raise the suspicion of migraine (Table 9.3). It is remarkable that profound changes in cerebral blood may be taking place during visual blurring in the early stages of migraine, since bilateral reductions in brain blood flow have now been seen with PET.[7]

Migraine with aura
From time to time patients with migraine aura (previously called classical migraine) are referred to ophthalmologists. This may be simply inappropriate or due to the aura being somewhat atypical. Migraine aura is generally visual in nature and may consist of bright flashing lights (photopsia), or jagged lines (fortification spectra) which have the key feature of moving slowly across the

175

Table 9.3   Simplified diagnostic criteria for migraine

Repeated attacks of headache last 4–72 hours which have these features:

at least 2 of:	*at least 1 of*:
• unilateral pain	• nausea/vomiting
• throbbing pain	• photophobia and phonophobia
• aggravation by movement	
• moderate or severe intensity	

Source: International Headache Society Guidelines[4]

visual field in contrast to the visual disturbances of cerebrovascular disease which have a rapid time course. Patients with the typical slow march of symptoms,[8] and more particularly those with subsequent or associated headache, can generally be reassured that they have migraine and referred for management. Certainly migraine aura without headache, acephalgic migraine, is seen and can again have the typical slow march of symptoms which is very reassuring. Some patients with visual aura will have more rapid onset disturbance and this requires more urgent attention to consider the differential diagnosis of transient ischaemic attacks. Ideally, a physician or neurologist should see these patients as soon as practicable.

Visual disturbance with eye pain

Pain in or around the eye is a common feature of retrobulbar neuritis and may be seen prior to visual disturbance. The pain may radiate over the frontal region with the visual disturbance varying from visual blurring to profound loss. The visual loss consists of a central scotoma and impaired colour vision. When there is optic disc swelling, papillitis, the relative loss of vision when compared to papilloedema associated with raised intracranial pressure is a very helpful clinical pointer. The most common cause of retrobulbar neuritis is demyelination. The likelihood of developing multiple sclerosis has been clarified somewhat in a recent study that followed patients with optic neuritis for 5 years. The risk of developing clinically definite multiple sclerosis ranged from 16% in 202 patients with no changes on MRI at the time of presentation to 51% of the 89 patients who had three or more lesions on MRI.[9] The likelihood of developing multiple sclerosis was unaffected by whether patients were treated with intravenous or oral steroids. In 28% of patients optic neuritis recurred in either eye. At 5 years the visual outcome was the same whether the patients had been treated with intravenous or oral steroids.[10] One might argue that only patients with marked visual loss, pain and lesions on MRI should be treated with intravenous steroids to try to reduce future disease activity, but otherwise oral steroids (prednisolone 1 mg/kg/day for 14 days) is an adequate treatment.

Visual disturbance with headache in the elderly

This section is deliberately highlighted to place emphasis on the issue of giant cell (temporal) arteritis which is an important problem, particularly in the elderly. Giant cell arteritis is predominantly a disease of patients over 50 years of age, with a prevalence of 133 per 100 000 in those over 50 rising to 843 per 100 000 in those over 80 years of age. Females are more affected than males.[11] The clinical picture often includes headache, with this being the presenting feature in half of the patients. The headache may be bilateral or unilateral and, although often temporal or bitemporal, may be generalised, so a high degree of suspicion must be held for the condition in the elderly. Sudden loss of vision may be a presenting feature in up to 23% of cases.[12] Other features of the illness include a low grade fever and muscle or joint pains. The inflammation may involve the posterior ciliary artery to cause visual disturbance including blindness. If there is involvement of the oculomotor nerve diplopia may be a presenting feature.

A high index of suspicion in the elderly should lead to an ESR measurement, which ranged in Koorey's cases from 40 to 140 mm/hour.[12] A normal ESR can be found with active disease,[13] so that a biopsy must be arranged immediately. The biopsy is positive in about half of the cases,[14] probably due to skip lesions.[15] The positive biopsy will demonstrate a thickened arterial wall and intima, with loss of the elastic lamina and infiltration of the media by round cells and giant cells. Treatment should not be delayed for a biopsy as vision is threatened; when the diagnosis is made, treatment should be instigated with either prednisolone 75 mg orally or methylprednisolone 500 mg intravenously in immediate consultation with a neurologist or general physician. The prognosis for patients with this condition may be poor if not handled adequately,

(a)

(b)

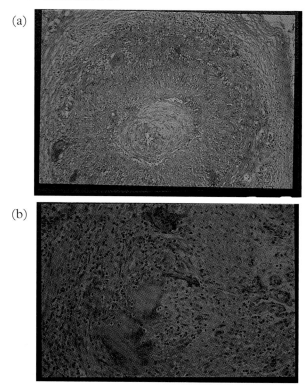

Figure 9.1 Low (a) and high (b) power photomicrographs of a temporal artery biopsy showing luminal obliteration, inflammatory infiltrate, and multinucleate giant cells (H&E stain).

with 44 out of 90 patients presenting to Moorfields Eye Hospital having visual loss.[16]

9.3 Headache or facial pain without visual disturbance

Although it would seem odd, many patients are referred for ophthalmological assessment who have no visual disturbance but simply headache. It is useful in this context to bear in mind that most of these patients with headache will not, provided they have no systemic illness, have any serious cause for headache (Table 9.1). From a neurological viewpoint it is helpful if the ophthalmologist checks for refractive errors, which will reassure

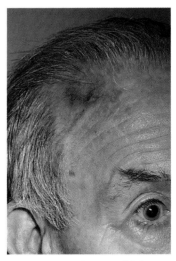

Figure 9.2 Prominent (pulseless and tender) superficial temporal artery with overlying ischaemic necrosis of skin in a patient with giant cell arteritis.

the patients with primary headache and make it easier to manage them later, and then parse the patients into two groups, those with immediate urgent problems and those without. With reference to Table 9.2, one can determine whether the patient has a potentially serious problem and make appropriate referral. The two major issues are sudden onset severe headache and persistent dull headache (tumour).

Head pain with eye signs but normal vision

The combination of head pain, particularly in the distribution of the ophthalmic division of the trigeminal nerve, with Horner's syndrome has been called Raeder's paratrigeminal neuralgia and has been reviewed by Mokri.[17] This term in essence describes a syndrome with several causes and draws attention to the anatomy of the sympathetic innervation of the eye. Third order sympathetic neurones from the cervical sympathetic chain pass up the common carotid artery and at the carotid bifurcation those involved in facial sweating and flushing continue by passing rostrally with the external carotid artery.[18] Fibres destined to innervate the pupil, levator of the eyelid, and the medial portion of the frontal scalp pass rostral with the internal carotid artery so that lesions of that internal

179

Table 9.4   Important urgent investigations in the headache patient

Presentation	Investigation	Possible pathology
Sudden onset headache		
with neck stiffness	Brain CT	Subarachnoid haemorrhage
	LP	Meningitis
without neck stiffness	Brain CT	Colloid cyst third ventricle
	MRA	Intracranial aneurysm
	MRI	Carotid or vertebral dissection
New headache in the elderly	ESR	Giant cell arteritis
New or changing headache	Brain CT	Tumour
		Idiopathic intracranial hypertension

carotid distal to the bifurcation and up to the cavernous sinus will produce an ocular (post-ganglionic) sympathetic deficit – Horner's syndrome – which spares facial sweating except for a small part of the medial aspect of the forehead. Pain in this setting indicates involvement of the trigeminal nerve and is usually referred to the ophthalmic division. Lesions such as dissection of the internal carotid, aneurysm, inflammation, trauma or neoplasm impinging on the vessel will then produce this syndrome and require referral and investigation. A sudden onset of the problem requires consideration of arterial dissection and should be promptly referred for neurological assessment.

Ophthalmodynia

Sudden stabbing pain in the eye has been described as "ophthalmodynia periodica". Lansche[19] reported that over 60% of patients with this syndrome were migraine sufferers. This author has not personally seen this syndrome and is unaware of any sinister cause. One wonders if it is a cousin of idiopathic jabbing or stabbing headaches,[4] which are common in patients with migraine. A treatment trial with indomethacin would be useful and interesting.[20]

9.4   Conclusion

The ophthalmologist may be faced with a wide range of clinical challenges from the somewhat introspective individual with some mild visual blurring and little else, through to a sudden onset headache with mild visual disturbance that is a sentinel bleed of a leaking aneurysm. Some conditions must be responded to immediately (Table 9.4) and others can be more gradually dealt with, and indeed in the largest part those with headache problems can be referred on to neurologists for further diagnosis and management. It is always a pleasure to see a referral from an ophthalmologist since patients have been reassured that their eyes are normal, which is often a step towards explaining the nature and management of primary headache syndromes.

1 Lance JW, Goadsby PJ. *Mechanism and management of headache* (6th edn). Oxford: Butterworth–Heinemann, 1998.
2 Goadsby PJ, Silberstein SD, eds. *Headache*. New York: Butterworth–Heinemann, 1997. (Asbury A, Marsden CD, eds. *Blue Books in Practical Neurology*, vol. 17.)
3 Rassmussen BK. Epidemiology of headache. *Cephalalgia* 1995;15: 45–68.
4 The Headache Classification Committee of the International Headache Society. Classification and diagnostic criteria for headache disorders, cranial neuralgias and facial pain. *Cephalalgia* 1988;8(Suppl 7):1–96.
5 Lyle TK. Ophthalmological headaches. In: Vinken PJ, Bruyn GW, eds. *Handbook of clinical neurology*, vol. 5. Amsterdam: North Holland, 1968:204–7.
6 Waters WE. Headache and the eye. A community study. *Lancet* 1970; ii:1–4.
7 Weiller C, May A, Limmroth V *et al.* Brain stem activation in spontaneous human migraine attacks. *Nature Med* 1995;1:658–60.
8 Lashley KS. Patterns of cerebral integration indicated by the scotomas of migraine. *Arch Neurol Psychiatry* 1941;46:331–9.
9 Optic Neuritis Study Group. The five-year risk of MS after optic neuritis. *Neurology* 1997;49:1404–13.
10 Optic Neuritis Study Group. Visual function 5 years after optic neuritis. *Arch Ophthalmol* 1997;115:1545–52.
11 Huston KA, Hunder GG, Lie JT, Kennedy RH, Elveback LR. Temporal arteritis. A 25 year epidemiologic, clinical and pathologic study. *Ann Intern Med* 1978;88:127–32.
12 Koorey DJ. Cranial arteritis. A twenty year review of cases. *Med J Aust* 1984;14:143–7.
13 Kansu T, Corbett JJ, Savino P, Schatz NJ. Giant cell arteritis with normal sedimentation rate. *Arch Neurol* 1977;34:624–5.
14 Murray TJ. Temporal arteritis. *J Am Geriatric Soc* 1977;25:450–3.
15 Klein RG, Campbell RJ, Hunder GG, Carney JA. Skip lesions in temporal arteritis. *Mayo Clin Proc* 1976;51:504–10.
16 Graham E, Holland A, Avery A, Ross Russell RW. Prognosis in giant-cell arteritis. *Br Med J* 1981;282:269–71.
17 Mokri B. Raeder's paratrigeminal neuralgia. Original concept and subsequent deviations. *Arch Neurol* 1982;39:395–9.

18 Drummond PD, Lance JW. Facial flushing and sweating mediated by a sympathetic nervous system. *Brain* 1987;**110**:793–803.
19 Lansche RK. Ophthalmodynia periodica. *Headache* 1964;**4**:247–9.
20 Mathew NT. Indomethacin-responsive headache syndromes. *Headache* 1981;**21**:147–50.

10: Disorders of pupillary function

FD BREMNER

Pupil abnormalities rarely have significant impact on visual function and so do not attract much attention from the busy clinician. However, as an aid to diagnosis the pupil has a central role to play in neuro-ophthalmology. Examination of the size and reactions of the pupil provides unique and objective information regarding function in many parts of the nervous system, including the parasympathetic and sympathetic pathways, the anterior visual pathways, and the brain stem. A full pupil evaluation takes only a few minutes to perform, requires no specialised equipment and in most cases can provide the diagnosis without the need for further investigation.

Before discussing disorders of pupillary function it is first necessary to understand the normal pupil. Pupil size is determined by the interaction of two opposing forces in the iris – the sphincter muscle (under parasympathetic control) and the dilator muscle (under sympathetic control). The parasympathetic supply is a two-neurone chain: the cell bodies of the preganglionic neurone lie within visceral midline nuclei (anteromedian and Edinger–Westphal) in the mesencephalon. Their axons join with the motor fibres of the oculomotor nerve, where they lie superficially and are susceptible to compressive injury, then leave within the orbit to terminate in the ciliary ganglion. The postganglionic fibres emerge as the short ciliary nerves passing forwards in the suprachoroidal space to reach the iris. The sympathetic supply is a three-neurone chain: the first order (central) neurone starts in the posterior

183

hypothalamus and descends uncrossed through the lateral part of the brain stem to terminate in the ciliospinal centre of Budge and Waller (level C8–T2). The second order (preganglionic) neurone leaves the spinal cord in the white rami communicantes and ascends in the sympathetic chain to terminate in the superior cervical ganglion. From here the third order (postganglionic) neurone follows the internal carotid artery intracranially, joining the abducens nerve and then the ophthalmic division of the trigeminal nerve before entering the orbit and passing forward to the iris dilator muscle in the long ciliary nerves.

The size and reactivity of the pupil are determined by a number of factors. These include alertness (setting the supranuclear inhibitory tone on the parasympathetic nuclei in the midbrain), emotions (psychic influences acting via the limbic system on the hypothalamus), accommodation (through the near triad synkinesis), and age (the pupils are largest in adolescents and progressively smaller thereafter). As a result there is significant variation in pupil size from moment to moment and in different people. Moreover the two pupils are often not the same size. The hallmarks of this physiological anisocoria are that it is similar when measured under light or dark conditions, it varies over time (it may even reverse) and the reactions to light or a near target are brisk and normal; these features should be contrasted with anisocoria due to parasympathetic or sympathetic block.

In this chapter pupillary disorders have been classified according to whether they principally affect the light reflex pathway (afferent, central or efferent defects) or the sympathetic pathway (Horner's syndrome).

10.1   Light reflex: afferent defects

In general, lesions of the afferent limb of the light reflex pathway do not affect the *size* of the pupils. For example, if one eye is blind then the sizes of both pupils are determined by the amount of light entering the other eye. If both eyes are blind then central factors such as arousal and accommodative effort determine whether the pupils are larger, smaller or the same size as in normal eyes. Afferent defects may only be detected by observing the *reactions* of the pupil to light.

Clinically this is assessed with the swinging light test where a flashlight is rapidly alternated between the two eyes and the pupil reactions compared. This test is best performed in dim light conditions using an intense stimulus (such as the beam from an indirect ophthalmoscope) allowing enough time for the pupils to equilibrate with the bright light (1–2 seconds) but not so long that the retinal pigment is bleached (>3 seconds). The test is valid even when only one pupil is functioning. With unilateral or asymmetric afferent defects the pupils react less to light shone in the worse eye (Marcus Gunn pupil). In the mildest cases, this relative afferent pupillary defect (RAPD) is suggested by asymmetry of the pupillary escape ("escape" is pupillary redilatation *before* the stimulus is withdrawn, a normal phenomenon which is exaggerated if there is an afferent defect). With more significant asymmetry the pupils dilate when the flashlight is swung from the better eye to the worse eye and constrict when the flashlight is swung back to the better eye. If there is no afferent function remaining then neither pupil will react to light shone in the affected eye ("amaurotic" pupils). The RAPD can be classified clinically as escape–mild– moderate–marked and quantified for research purposes using neutral density filters or infrared video pupillography.

The presence of an RAPD indicates asymmetry in the afferent signals from the two eyes. It is most commonly associated with *retinal* or *optic nerve* disease. It is rare for *preretinal* disease to be so severe as to significantly affect the pupils: in cases where there is a poor view of the fundus due to advanced cataract or vitreous haemorrhage it is unwise to ascribe the presence of an RAPD to these media opacities. Intriguingly, infrared video pupillography can demonstrate afferent pupil defects due to *retrochiasmal* disease, including suprageniculate lesions[1,2] but these rarely produce a clinically detectable RAPD. The extent of the RAPD broadly correlates with the degree of loss of visual field. It should be remembered that the presence of an RAPD may not mean that the "better" eye is a *normal* eye, merely that it is less affected. Occasionally bilateral afferent defects are found which are truly symmetrical and present as pupils with poor light reactions, no RAPD, and normal near reactions.[3]

10.2 Light reflex: central defects

With midbrain lesions vision is preserved but the patient shows bilateral symmetrical pupillary abnormalities and other signs of brain stem dysfunction. The two main patterns of abnormality seen are Parinaud's syndrome and Argyll Robertson pupils. Parinaud's syndrome (also known as dorsal midbrain, pretectal, Sylvian aqueduct or Koerber–Salus–Elschnig syndrome) is characterised by *large regular* pupils which constrict briskly to an accommodative target but poorly if at all to light ("light–near dissociation"). Associated findings include vertical gaze deficit, convergence–retraction nystagmus, Collier's sign (lid retraction), and skew deviation. This pattern of deficits implies a lesion affecting the posterior commissure and pretectal nuclei and is most commonly associated with pineal region tumours, hydrocephalus or intrinsic lesions of the dorsal midbrain.[4]

Argyll Robertson (AR) pupils are rarely seen nowadays. They show similar light–near dissociation but are *small and irregular*, dilating poorly in darkness and often showing an attenuated response to topical mydriatic agents. These features suggest interruption of the central inhibitory fibres ventral to the aqueduct (Figure 10.1), although a corresponding focal lesion has yet to be demonstrated. AR pupils are usually considered pathognomonic of tertiary syphilis but "pseudo-AR" pupils showing many or all of the above features have been described in a number of other conditions including diabetes mellitus, multiple sclerosis, encephalitis, and myotonic dystrophy (see review by Loewenfeld[5]). It should be noted that other patterns of pupillary abnormality are occasionally found in tertiary syphilis including spastic miosis (no near or light reactions) and "inverse-AR" pupils (absent near reaction with preserved light reaction); in practice it is wise to test for syphilis in all cases of an unexplained central pupillary defect.[5]

10.3 Light reflex: efferent defects

Parasympathetic block may be preganglionic (the unreactive pupil) or postganglionic (the "tonic" pupil).[6] Preganglionic block is characterised by a large, unreactive pupil, absent accommodation and paresis of some or all of the other muscles supplied by the oculomotor nerve. Isolated pupil involvement without external ophthalmoplegia can occur and usually indicates a *surgical* (compressive) cause (but beware basal meningitis). In the acute phase the pupil will not constrict to dilute pilocarpine (0.1%); in longstanding cases disuse atrophy of the postganglionic fibres may lead to secondary "denervation" supersensitivity. Parasellar lesions compressing the oculomotor nerve often cause aberrant

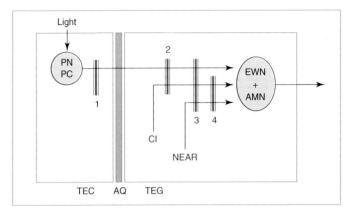

Figure 10.1 Schematic diagram of the midbrain pathways involved in different central pupillary disorders. Pathways shown serve the light reaction (PN, pretectal nuclei; PC, posterior commissure), the near reaction and the central inhibitory fibres (mostly from the reticular activating system) which suppress the high spontaneous rate of discharge from neurones in the Edinger–Westphal (EWN) and anteromedian (AMN) nuclei. Lesions at various sites within the tectum (TEC) and tegmentum (TEG) give rise to: (1) Parinaud's syndrome; (2) Argyll Robertson pupils; (3) spastic miosis; (4) inverse-AR pupils. AQ, sylvian aqueduct.

regeneration over time: the commonest synkinesis is with medial rectus motor units producing miosis during adduction and convergence movements.

In the *acute* phase postganglionic block is characterised by a large, unreactive pupil and cycloplegia which is indistinguishable from a preganglionic block. However, with time there is aberrant regeneration of these postganglionic fibres and the pupil exhibits "tonic" behaviour (the Adie's pupil): there is light–near dissociation and the pupil is much slower to constrict and to redilate after a light or near stimulus (sometimes minutes). At the slit-lamp the reinnervation is seen to be patchy with areas of sectoral palsy leading to "streaming" and "vermiform" movements (note: the iris does not transilluminate in contrast to cases of herpes zoster or angle closure glaucoma where the damage is ischaemic). Accommodation recovers quickly but the pupillary abnormalities persist with gradual miosis over time: in some cases the pupil ends up smaller than in the fellow eye. Denervation supersensitivity is readily demonstrated within days of the initial damage using 0.1% pilocarpine.

The tonic pupil is most commonly found in Adie's syndrome, a benign idiopathic condition which typically affects young women in their third to fifth decades. It is unilateral in 80–90% of cases and may present with sudden blurring of vision, photophobia, anisocoria or without symptoms as an incidental finding. Pain is not a feature. The diagnosis is made by demonstrating reduced deep tendon reflexes (especially knee and ankle) and excluding other ocular and orbital causes of a tonic pupil. A small proportion of these patients have been reported as also having patchy hypohidrosis from involvement of sudomotor fibres (Ross's syndrome). Other causes of a tonic pupil are much rarer but include orbital injuries, orbital surgery, orbital tumours, herpes zoster, extensive panretinal photocoagulation or cryotherapy.

Mimics of parasympathetic blockade abound. Many congenital or acquired lesions of the iris can lead to a large, unreactive pupil and should be excluded by careful examination with the slit lamp (sphincter ruptures in cases of trauma can be easily missed and are best demonstrated by retroilluminating the pupil margin). The use of atropine-like drugs may not be offered in the history but is suggested by a total internal ophthalmoplegia without denervation supersensitivity, and with normal ocular motility. In doubtful cases the passage of time will clarify the situation.

Neuro-imaging is mandatory to investigate preganglionic block since structural lesions account for a significant proportion of pupil-involving oculomotor nerve palsies. Postganglionic block rarely needs investigation. The management of the parasympathetic block should be directed at the symptoms. For accommodative paresis, reading glasses or bifocals may help. For troublesome glare, dilute pilocarpine drops (used sparingly) can be very effective but the clinician needs to avoid triggering accommodative spasm through ciliary muscle supersensitivity. Many patients with Adie's syndrome require only reassurance that the condition is limited and benign.

10.4   Sympathetic defects: Horner's syndrome

Patients with unilateral Horner's syndrome (oculosympathetic paresis) may complain of ptosis or anisocoria but often it is an incidental finding: it should be specifically looked for in all patients complaining of unexplained arm or head pain. The affected pupil is small, with increased anisocoria in dim conditions, and sluggish redilatation when the light is switched off. Additionally, because sympathetic innervation is important for the early development of iris pigmentation, there may be heterochromia iridis in congenital

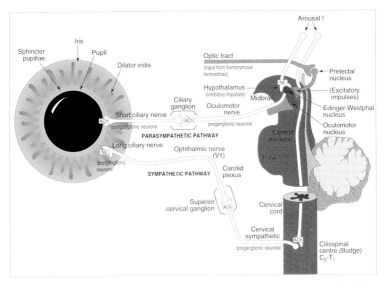

Figure 10.2   The parasympathetic and sympathetic innervation of the iris muscles. From the CNS to the effector muscles there are always two neurones (preganglionic and postganglionic). This is also true for the ciliary muscle that controls accommodation. Both ganglia (ciliary and superior cervical) are cholinergic, but the sympathetic neuro-effector junction is adrenergic. Notice that the inhibitory fibres to the sphincter nucleus (Edinger–Westphal) are also adrenergic, so that centrally and peripherally noradrenaline acts to dilate the pupil.

or perinatal Horner's. Other features of Horner's syndrome include mild ptosis, elevation of the lower lid (giving rise to apparent enophthalmos), conjunctival injection, and ocular hypotony. With preganglionic lesions the ipsilateral skin may feel warmer and drier due to interruption of the sudomotor supply; postganglionic lesions distal to the carotid bifurcation do not cause facial anhydrosis apart from a small patch of skin above the supraorbital notch which is supplied by sudomotor fibres travelling with the internal carotid artery.

The pharmacological abnormalities in Horner's are summarised in Table 10.1. Denervation supersensitivity to dilute phenylephrine is sometimes but not invariably present. A more reliable test for Horner's is 4% cocaine which increases the basal sympathetic tone in the normal iris dilator muscle by preventing noradrenaline re-uptake. In Horner's the affected pupil has such a low basal sympathetic tone that little or no mydriasis occurs: a post-cocaine anisocoria greater than 0.8 mm is highly diagnostic of

189

Horner's syndrome.[7] Further classification of Horner's as pre- or postganglionic may be achieved with the use of 1% hydroxy-amphetamine. This releases noradrenaline from *intact* post-ganglionic neurones and will therefore dilate normal pupils and pupils with preganglionic Horner's of recent onset. In longstanding preganglionic Horner's the test is difficult to interpret since there is often a degree of disuse atrophy of the third order neurone. For all of these pharmacological tests a single drop only should be given since repeated instillation leads to dosing confusion. It is necessary to allow a wash-out interval of 48 hours between the cocaine test and the hydroxyamphetamine test.

Table 10.1   Summary of responses to topical 1% phenylephrine (PHE), 4% cocaine (COC) and 1% hydroxyamphetamine (AMP) in normal pupils and in Horner's syndrome

Pupil/lesion	Duration	1% PHE	4% COC	1% AMP
Normal		−	+	+
Horner's/preganglionic	Recent	±	−	+
Horner's/preganglionic	Longstanding	±	−	−
Horner's/postganglionic		±	−	−

Responses found are: +, dilates; ±, sometimes dilates; −, no response.

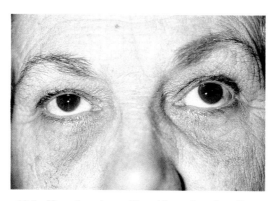

Figure 10.3   Horner's syndrome. Note right ptosis and pupillary miosis.

Horner's syndrome is of little functional significance regarding vision, a point which often needs to be stated clearly to reassure the anxious patient. However, its importance lies in the nature of the pathology which caused it. Horner's syndrome can be produced by lesions anywhere along the lengthy course of the sympathetic

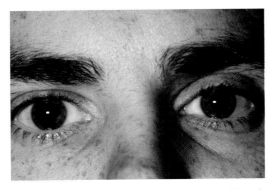

Figure 10.4 Anisocoria may require very careful evaluation: this patient had a left Horner's plus a right Holmes Adie pupil. Note slightly irregular right pupil margin.

supply to the eye. The first order ("central") neurone may be involved in brain stem (pontine infarction, lateral medullary syndrome, multiple sclerosis) or cervical cord (trauma, tumours, syringomyelia) lesions and is invariably associated with other signs of axial pathology. The second order ("preganglionic") neurone is susceptible to chest (Pancoast's tumour, cervical rib, surgery) or neck (trauma, tumours, surgery) disease and may be isolated or associated only with arm pain. In children any preganglionic Horner's without a history of birth trauma, regardless of iris pigmentation, requires urgent imaging to exclude a neuroblastoma. In adults, acquired preganglionic Horner's usually needs further investigation since a small proportion of these patients harbour an unsuspected malignancy. Isolated lesions of the third order ("postganglionic") neurone are usually benign, may be associated with episodic pain in a trigeminal distribution (Raeder's paratrigeminal syndrome) and require no further investigation. The clinician should be wary, however, of the acute onset postganglionic Horner's which presents with constant and severe jaw and head pain in a patient with systemic vascular disease or significant neck trauma: these patients require urgent magnetic resonance angiography (arteriography is contraindicated) to exclude carotid dissection.

Bilateral Horner's syndrome is found in a number of autonomic neuropathies including diabetes mellitus, progressive autonomic failure, and amyloidosis. It is often missed clinically because the signs are symmetrical in the two eyes. The diagnosis can be

191

confirmed with cocaine or using infrared video pupillography to quantify the redilatation lag.

Acknowledgement

Figure 10.2 is reproduced from Rosen ES, Thompson HS, Cumming WJ, Eustace P. *Neuro-ophthalmology*. London: Mosby, 1997.

1 Hamann K-U, Hellner KA, Müller-Jensen A, Zschocke S. Videopupillographic and VER investigations in patients with congenital and acquired lesions of the optic radiation. *Ophthalmologica* 1979;**178**: 348–56.
2 Thompson HS, Corbett JJ. Asymmetry of pupillomotor input. *Eye* 1991;**5**:36–9.
3 Thompson HS, Corbett JJ, Cox TA. How to measure the relative afferent pupillary defect. *Surv Ophthalmol* 1981;**26**:39–42.
4 Thompson HS, Kardon RH. Pretectal pupillary defects: editorial comment. *J Clin Neuro-Ophthalmol* 1991;**11**:173–4.
5 Loewenfeld IE. The Argyll Robertson pupil 1869–1969: a critical survey of the literature. *Surv Ophthalmol* 1969;**14**:199–299.
6 Loewenfeld IE, Thompson HS. Mechanism of tonic pupil. *Ann Neurol* 1981;**10**:275–6.
7 Kardon RH, Denison CE, Brown CK *et al.* Critical evaluation of the cocaine test in the diagnosis of Horner's syndrome. *Arch Ophthalmol* 1990;**108**:384–7.

11: Eyelid and facial disorders

JF ACHESON

11.1 Synopsis of anatomy of the facial nerve

The neural pathways for the muscles of facial expression arise in the motor cortex, and are relayed via the facial nucleus in the pons to the facial (VIIth cranial) nerve. The peripheral facial nerve passes through the subarachnoid space (in the cerebellopontine angle), and the temporal bone before forming an extracranial segment to reach the face.

Supranuclear pathways

The cortical control for voluntary facial movements lies in the precentral gyrus of the frontal cerebral cortex. Supranuclear fibres are carried by the corticobulbar tract to the genu of the internal capsule and then to the facial nucleus in the pons via the cerebral peduncles. The portion of the facial nucleus supplying the muscles of the upper face (frontalis, orbicularis, oculi) receives corticobulbar fibres from both cerebral hemispheres, but the portion supplying the lower face receives fibres from the contralateral side only. Thus a unilateral hemisphere lesion will cause a contralateral weakness of the lower face only, while a lower motor neurone facial weakness will involve the entire face on the same side.

Reflex and automatic facial movements are regulated by the extrapyramidal system with the result that patients with this group of disorders demonstrate either a lack of facial expression, as in Parkinson's disease, or the involuntary facial movements which characterise Meige's syndrome of blepharospasm and orofacial dystonia among other conditions.

Pons

In the pons, the facial nucleus is located in the ventrolateral angle of the tegmentum. The motor axons pass dorsally, looping around the abducens nerve to form the pontine genu in the floor of the fourth ventricle before exiting the brain stem laterally together with the vestibulo-acoustic (VIIIth) nerve and the nervus intermedius. The nervus intermedius comprises visceral efferent fibres passing from the superior salivary nucleus to the sublingual, submandibular, and lacrimal glands, together with special visceral afferent fibres serving taste sensation in the anterior two-thirds of the tongue and somatic sensory afferents from the posterior wall of the external auditory meatus.

Cerebellopontine angle

The facial nerve, nervus intermedius and the VIIIth cranial nerve share a meningeal covering on exit from the pons before entering the lateral pontine cistern. The fibres of the nervus intermedius are loosely joined to the motor facial nerve near the entry to the internal acoustic meatus in the cerebellopontine angle and the anterior inferior cerebellar artery may loop between the VIIth and VIIIth nerves at this point. Mass lesions in the cerebellopontine angle frequently impair function of the nervus intermedius resulting in abnormalities of tearing, taste, and submandibular saliva flow, and of the vestibulo-acoustic nerve with hearing and balance loss, in addition to causing facial weakness. Large tumours also cause defects of the Vth, IXth and Xth nerves (for example cholesteatoma, vestibular schwannoma, meningioma). In addition, hyperkinetic disorders may be attributed to vascular compression of the facial nerve root as it crosses the subarachnoid space.

Temporal bone

In a Z-shaped course through the temporal bone, the facial nerve incorporates labyrinthine, tympanic, and mastoid segments. The labyrinthine segment includes the geniculate ganglion, serving the afferent fibres of the nervus intermedius. The greater superficial petrosal nerve leaves the facial nerve at this point to synapse at the spheno-palatine ganglion and eventually reach the lacrimal gland via the zygomatico-temporal branch of the Vth nerve (V2) and the lacrimal nerve (V1). Lacrimal fibres also reach their destination via branches of the Vth and IXth cranial nerves. Turning a right-angle posteriorly at the genu, the facial nerve passes through the middle ear (tympanic segment) giving off a branch to the stapedius muscle and then turns inferiorly (mastoid segment) to exit the temporal bone at the stylomastoid foramen. The chorda tympani is the terminal branch of the nervus intermedius and usually arises from the mastoid segment to convey secretor motor fibres to the sublingual and submandibular glands, special sensory afferents from the anterior tongue, and somatic sensory afferents from the posterior wall of the external auditory meatus.

Extracranial segment

After giving off branches to muscles of the anterior triangle of the neck, the main trunk of the facial nerve enters the parotid gland, bifurcates and then divides again in a variety of patterns to form temporal, zygomatic, buccal, mandibular and cervical branches. Intercommunications between these branches and fibres to the salivary glands account for the aberrant regeneration syndromes of facial synkinesis and crocodile tears which may follow facial nerve injury.

11.2 Synopsis of anatomy and physiology of the eyelids

The levator palpebrae superioris is the principle muscle involved in opening the upper lid and for maintaining normal lid position – accessory roles are played by the frontalis and Müller's muscles. Both the levator and superior rectus have a common origin from the lesser wing of the sphenoid bone at the orbital apex. About 1 cm behind the orbital septum it ends as a membranous expansion, or aponeurosis which spreads out to attach to the tarsal plate, the orbital septum, and the suspensory ligaments. Müller's muscle is composed of a thin band of smooth muscle fibres lying on the inferior surface of the levator and inserts on to the tarsal plate. The frontalis muscle acts as an indirect lid elevator by means of attachments to the orbicularis oculi muscle.

The tone of the levator palpebrae (LP) muscle is governed by both the corticobulbar and extrapyramidal systems which synapse with neurones of the levator nucleus in the oculomotor complex via the periaqueductal grey. Although the LP motor nucleus is unpaired, the premotor control of the LP is lateralised in part in the cortex, extrapyramidal system and rostral brain stem. The diffuse projections of the reticular activating system also influence eyelid opening and lid position reflects arousal levels. Within the oculomotor complex in the mesencephalon, the levator nucleus lies in the midline, caudally and dorsally sending fibres to join the other axons of each oculomotor nerve. The principle of equal innervation of yoked extraocular muscles (Hering's law) applies to the eyelids so that if one eyelid is ptotic, the other will retract as extra innervation flows to both sides. During normal fast and slow vertical eye movements the tonus of the levator is directly linked to that of the superior rectus so that the upper lids accurately follow the movements of the globe. During sleep and forced eyelid closure, however, the levator is inhibited as the superior rectus contracts (Bell's phenomenon).[1]

11.3   Facial weakness

Clinical assessment

Careful observation of the patient at rest often reveals a subtle facial weakness resulting in a flattened nasolabial fold and a wider palpebral aperture on the affected side. In supranuclear lesions, preservation of forehead frontalis function is typical due to bilateral cortical representation of these muscles. In other supranuclear disorders, there may be a dissociation between normal involuntary facial movements such as grimacing or blinking to a bright light and inability to perform voluntary movements. In infranuclear lesions, weakness of the orbicularis oculi muscle group becomes especially obvious on attempted eyelid closure, because the eye may stay open (lagophthalmos) and the palpebral-oculogyric reflex

(Bell's phenomenon) is preserved driving the eye upwards and outwards.[2]

Impaired ipsilateral taste function and tear secretion indicates that the lesion is peripheral to the facial nucleus. Tear secretion is important clinically not only because of the localising value of noting loss of function in fibres to the lacrimal gland via the greater superficial petrosal nerve and nervus intermedius, but also because of the increased risk of corneal ulceration and visual loss in facial palsy which results from incomplete lid closure when combined with deficient lubrication.

Table 11.1   The House classification system for reporting results of recovery from facial palsy[3]

Degree of injury	Grade	Definition
Normal	I	No abnormality
Mild dysfunction	II	Complete eyelid closure without effort
		Slight smile asymmetry
Moderate dysfunction	III	Obvious weakness on resting
		Brow ptosis
		Eyelid closure on effort
		Mouth movement with effort
Moderate–severe dysfunction	IV	Disfiguring weakness
		Incomplete eyelid closure
		Mouth asymmetry on maximal effort
		Synkinesis and mass movement
Severe dysfunction	V	Motion barely perceptible
		Synkinesis and mass movement absent
Total paralysis	VI	No movement and complete loss of tone

Causes of peripheral facial palsy

Intra-axial lesions

The facial nerve is involved in the dorsolateral pontine syndrome of Foville, comprising ipsilateral paralysis of abduction (or gaze palsy), lower motor neurone facial palsy, loss of taste in the anterior two-thirds of the tongue, Horner's syndrome, facial analgesia, and peripheral deafness. Partial forms are more frequent than the full syndrome. Facial weakness is also seen in paramedian and basal pontine lesions (Millard–Gubler syndrome) with additional ipsilateral abducens palsy and contralateral hemiplegia. Intrinsic pontine lesions are usually the result of infarction, haemorrhage, tumour or demyelination. Congenital facial palsy often arises at the level of the brain stem, referred to as the Möbius syndrome.

197

Peripheral lesions

Peripheral causes of facial palsy include herpes zoster cephalicus (geniculate zoster or Ramsay–Hunt syndrome), when there is severe pain in and around the ear. Vesicles may appear in the external auditory canal, and sometimes also on the face and neck and within the mouth. Other infectious and immune-related neuropathies which cause facial weakness include postinfectious polyradiculopathy (Guillain–Barré syndrome), infectious mononucleosis, Lyme disease, complicated otitis media (Gradinego's syndrome), leprosy, and syphilis.

Additional causes include trauma (basal skull fractures, neurosurgery), tumours in the cerebellopontine angle and facial neuromas, metastatic deposits or carcinomatous meningitis, and sarcoidosis.

Finally, metabolic diseases (acute porphyria) and myopathic processes (myasthenia gravis, myotonic dystrophy, botulism) need to be excluded before a diagnosis of idiopathic acute facial palsy (Bell's palsy) can be made. In Bell's palsy, subjective complaints of pain and facial numbness are frequent, as are recurrent episodes. Dysacusis and abnormalities of taste and salivary secretion indicate a lesion of the tympanomastoid portion of the facial nerve within the temporal bone. There is an association between Bell's palsy and both diabetes and pregnancy, and a positive family history may be present.

Ophthalmic aspects of the management of facial palsy

The most pressing aspect of the care of a patient with facial palsy is protection of the eye. Lagophthalmos results in corneal drying and epithelial ulceration with the risk of blindness from infective keratitis and corneal vascularisation. The risk is increased because of concomitant tear film insufficiency, and most of all when there is additional loss of function in the ophthalmic division of the trigeminal nerve causing loss of sensation and neurotrophic corneal changes. The use of ocular lubricants alone is often inadequate and lid taping is mandatory when the patient is asleep or unconscious. When the corneal epithelium ulcerates in spite of these measures, a temporary ptosis induced by botulinum toxin levator chemodenervation may be valuable to allow time for spontaneous recovery of facial function or for the planning of a definitive tarsorrhaphy. Nowadays oculoplastic surgery can be used

Table 11.2   Causes of facial nerve disorders

Cause	%
Bell's palsy (idiopathic)	53
Trauma	21
Accidental	
Iatrogenic and surgical	
Herpes zoster (Ramsay–Hunt syndrome)	8
Tumours	7
Acoustic neuroma	
Facial neuroma	
Non-Hodgkin's lymphoma	
Carcinomatous meningitis	
Infections and inflammation	4
Polyradiculopathy	
Infectious mononucleosis	
Lyme disease	
Middle ear infection	
Basal meningitis	
Sarcoidosis	
Melkersson–Rosenthal syndrome	
Birth (congenital and acquired)	3
Hemifacial spasm	2
CNS disease (axial lesions)	1
Other	2
Acute porphyrias	
Myasthenia gravis	
Botulism	
Myotonic dystrophy	
Progressive hemifacial atrophy	

Source: May M, Galetta S. The facial nerve and related disorders of the face. In: Glaser JS, ed. *Clinical Neuro-Ophthalmology*. Lippincott: Philadelphia, 1990:255

to achieve some degree of palpebral symmetry in unrecovered facial palsy, as well as to provide corneal protection. Available techniques include medial and lateral tarsorrhaphy, canthal slings, and procedures to lower the upper lid by retractor recession or by weighting the tarsus with gold implants. Facial nerve anastomosis, facial–hypoglossal nerve transfer and temporalis transfer may all play an additional role in rehabilitation.[4]

11.4   Hyperkinetic facial syndromes

Spontaneous anomalous facial movements may frequently present as an ophthalmic complaint. These include primary and secondary blepharospasm, hemifacial spasm, facial synkinesis following recovery from facial palsy, tonic contracture, and myokymia.

Blepharospasm

Essential (idiopathic) blepharospasm is a form of focal dystonia typically affecting patients in their 6th and 7th decades, more frequently women than men, which is characterised by involuntary and repetitive eyelid closure due to spasmodic contraction of the orbicularis oculi muscles in the absence of significant ocular pathology. It is usually bilateral and often progressive in severity. In many patients the movement disorder includes both blepharospasm and oromandibular dystonia (Breughel's syndrome or Meige's disease). In others blepharospasm arises as part of a generalised or secondary dystonia of which the causes include basal ganglia infarction, Wilson's disease, neuroleptic drugs, and progressive supranuclear palsy. The intensity of spasms may range from increased blinking caused by external stimuli (bright lights, wind), to mild noticeable inappropriate eyelid closure through to moderate spasms and severe, functionally incapacitating spasms.[5]

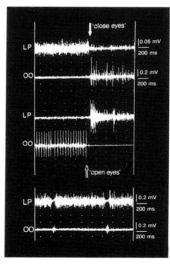

Figure 11.1   Simultaneous EMG traces recorded from orbicularis and levator muscles showing normal reciprocal innervation.

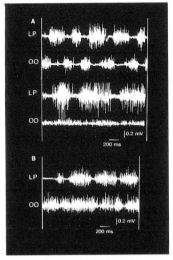

Figure 11.2   Dystonic co-contraction of orbicularis and levator muscles in a patient with blepharospasm.

In some individuals the levator inhibition is the dominant abnormality. Lid elevation may be accomplished after backward head thrusts, extensive frontalis action or by digital rubbing of the frontalis. This is often termed apraxia of eyelid opening.[6]

Pharmacological and biofeedback therapies are usually disappointing and surgical treatments including orbicularis stripping and facial nerve avulsion are only indicated in the last

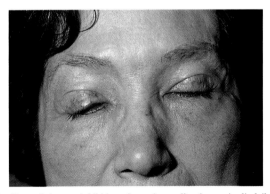

Figure 11.3   Dystonic levator inhibition: the patient suffers from episodic failure of normal voluntary eyelid opening.

201

resort. However, injections of the presynaptic blocking agent botulinum ("a gift from ophthalmology to neurology", Alan Scott) are useful. Botulinum is injected subcutaneously into the orbicularis oculi muscles with the result that most patients enjoy a significant reduction in facial spasms within a few days of injection and lasting for an average of 3 months. Longer term benefit is limited by axonal resprouting resulting in reinnervation of injected muscles but repeated injections are well tolerated. Patients with typical blepharospasm including depressed eyebrows and with obvious orbital orbicularis contraction respond better to botulinum toxin injections than those with no obvious contracture of the orbicularis. Application of botulinum into multiple sites in the orbicularis, especially the pretarsal portion, may be associated with better and less variable responses to treatment.[7]

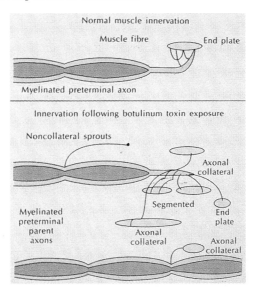

Figure 11.4   Regrowth of new axonal sprouts in orbicularis muscle following botulinum chemodenervation.

Hemifacial spasm

In hemifacial spasm unilateral periodic tonic and clonic facial contractions usually start around the eye and then, as the condition progresses, spasms may involve the whole face including the

202

Table 11.3   Assessment of visual disability in blepharospasm[8]

Category/description	Visual function
Blind	No effective function
Dependent	Needs assistance to move outside familiar environment
Independent (poor function)	Able to walk independently: unable to drive, read, watch television, severe photophobia
Independent (moderate function)	Limited practical function, eg cannot work, read
Inconvenienced	Intermittent interference; unable to drive; can work
Normal	

platysma muscle. In contrast to idiopathic blepharospasm, the involuntary movements occur in sleep as well as when the patient is awake. The differential diagnosis includes focal epilepsy, facial neuromyotonia, myokymia, and facial synkinesia. MR imaging of the posterior fossa may reveal extramedullary compressive lesions of the facial nerve including basilar aneurysm and tumours in the cerebellopontine angle. Many patients can be satisfactorily managed by using botulinum toxin injections to the affected muscles with repeated treatments as required: others find that night-time use of carbamazepine is adequate.[9]

Facial synkinesis

Following a VIIth nerve paresis, a patient may demonstrate ipsilateral involuntary narrowing of the palpebral aperture when other facial muscle groups are voluntarily moved. In a typical instance, mouth movements (orbicularis oris) whilst eating or smiling are associated with unwanted eye closure.

Botulinum toxin injections may offer temporary relief, given on the same basis as for the treatment of hemifacial spasm.

A further aberrant regeneration syndrome following facial nerve injury at or above the level of the geniculate ganglion is gustatory tearing (crocodile tears), where parasympathetic fibres supplying the salivary glands via the chorda tympani become misrouted with the result that the stimulus to salivate (food or the prospect of food) is inappropriately accompanied by ipsilateral tearing. A variety of anatomical mechanisms have been proposed: misrouting of visceromotor fibres from the chorda tympani to the greater

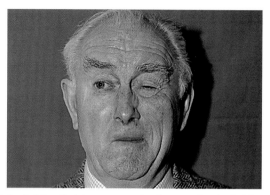

Figure 11.5 Left hemifacial spasm: note involvement of entire facial musculature.

superficial petrosal nerve and thence to the lacrimal gland, anomalous collateral sprouting of fibres from the glossopharyngeal nerve to the greater superficial petrosal nerve at the tympanic plexus, and proximal misrouting at the site of afferent and visceromotor fibres in the nervus intermedius. Transtympanic division of the tympanic branch of the glossopharyngeal nerve is probably the definitive surgical solution to an acquired gustolacrimal reflex following facial palsy. Vidian neurectomy in the pterygopalatine fossa may also help.

Facial myokymia

Facial myokymia is characterised by a fine fibrillary movement of the facial muscles in a unilateral intermittent pattern. A benign form is common, limited to the eyelids in a transient manner that is apparently exacerbated by anxiety or fatigue. More generalised involvement is associated with intrinsic brain stem lesions and with extramedullary compression, requiring formal evaluation. Occasionally there is additional facial contracture and paresis indicating an intrinsic pontine lesion rostral to the facial nucleus.

11.5 Ptosis

Neuropathic ptosis is usually the result of loss of function of the oculomotor nerve or the oculosympathetic pathway (infranuclear ptosis), but both supranuclear and nuclear forms are also seen.

204

Both unilateral and bilateral ptosis may occur in hemispheric lesions, usually following a stroke (cerebral ptosis).[10] One characteristic variant is the failure of initiation of eyelid opening which results from a transient failure to overcome levator inhibitory pathways. This is known as "apraxia of eyelid opening" and frequently full elevation of the upper lids can only be accomplished by a special manoeuvre such as thrusting the head backwards, or by massaging the brow.[11] Apraxia of eyelid opening is also a frequent feature of dystonic blepharospasm (see above).

Mesencephalic ptosis results from destructive or congenital lesions of the upper brain stem which involve the caudal portion of the oculomotor complex, or the floor of the IIIrd ventricle or rostral midbrain. Infranuclear ptosis may result from fascicular and peripheral lesions of the oculomotor nerve. Pupillary and extraocular muscle involvement is usual, but an isolated unilateral ptosis may arise in patients with intracranial aneurysm and intracavernous meningioma. In ptosis due to oculosympathetic paresis (Horner's syndrome) the abnormality is usually mild, there is an "upside down" ptosis of the lower lid due to involvement of the lower lid Müller's muscle and ipsilateral miosis.

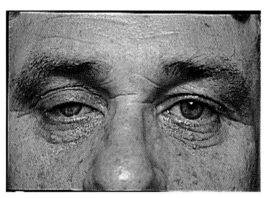

Figure 11.6   Right ptosis and iris heterochromia in early onset Horner's syndrome.

Ptosis arising from abnormalities at the neuromuscular junction and from myopathies may be congenital or acquired. Congenital ptosis occurs frequently and is usually due to maldevelopment of the levator muscle or its tendon. Unilateral and bilateral involvement may be seen: typically in addition to limitation of lid elevation on upgaze, there is limited depression on downgaze reflecting abnormal muscle relaxation. Acquired ptosis is seen in the mitochondrial cytopathies which cause chronic progressive external ophthalmoplegia, in myotonic dystrophy, in myasthenia and other neuromuscular junction diseases, and also following trauma, inflammation or infiltration of the levator or its tendon.

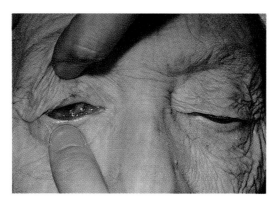

Figure 11.7   Severe myopathic ptosis: note paralytic lower lid ectropion on left eye and weak orbicularis function on attempted forced eyelid closure on right.

Disinsertion of the levator tendon results in involutional ptosis in the elderly, in long term contact lens wearers, and following various types of elective ocular surgery. In such cases the range of levator function is typically full, and the skin is indistinct and elevated. Diagnostic confusion is also caused by "pseudoptosis" arising when one eye is deviated downwards (hypotropic) or in enophthalmos and microphthalmos.

11.6   Eyelid retraction

Congenital causes of lid retraction include the Marcus Gunn phenomenon, in which there is paradoxic eyelid retraction evoked by jaw movement or swallowing. This is thought to represent a trigemino-oculomotor synkinesis, and is subdivided into internal pterygoid and external pterygoid forms. The external pterygoid form is the most frequent, in which there is a unilateral ptosis followed by lid elevation in association with the jaw moving to the opposite side or projecting forward. In the internal pterygoid form the lid elevates on closing the mouth or clenching the teeth.

Acquired eyelid retraction may arise in supranuclear lesions of the periaqueductal and dorsal midbrain regions. This is referred to as Collier's sign and may be seen in isolation or in association with the other features of Parinaud's syndrome (pupillary light–near dissociation, vertical gaze abnormalities, convergence–retraction nystagmus). Eyelid retraction is also seen in aberrant regeneration of the oculomotor nerve, when the lid elevates in association with elevation, depression or adduction of the involved eye. Primary aberrant regeneration of the IIIrd nerve is said to be a characteristic feature of intracavernous aneurysms and meningiomas. The commonest pattern observed is retraction of the lid on depression of the eye (pseudo-von Graefe's sign), but medial rectus contraction and adduction may also generate the same effect. When the fellow eye is ptotic, the upper lid may show abnormal retraction as a result of equal innervation flowing to each lid in an attempt to overcome a peripheral weakness on one side.

Myopathic processes cause abnormal lid elevation: maternal hyperthyroidism causes transient congenital lid retraction. In established dysthyroid eye disease, lid retraction may reflect hyperthyroidism with potentiation of the action of Müller's muscle, pathologic shortening of the levator muscle or overaction of the superior rectus–levator muscle complex in an attempt to overcome a pathologically shortened inferior rectus muscle.

Finally, the upper lids may be involved in nystagmus. Eyelid nystagmus on attempted convergence is associated with ill-defined cerebellar or brain stem damage.

1 Schmidtke K, Büttner-Ennever A. Nervous control of eyelid function. *Brain* 1992;**115**:227–47.
2 Francis IL, Loughread JA. Bell's phenomenon. A study of 508 patients. *Aust J Ophthalmol* 1984;**12**:15–21.
3 House JW. Facial nerve grading system. *Laryngoscope* 1983;**93**: 1056–69.
4 Sadiq SA. Downes RN. A clinical algorithm for the management of facial nerve palsy from an oculoplastic perspective. *Eye* 1998;**12**(2): 219–23.
5 Beradelli A, Rothwell JC, Day BL, Marsden CD. Pathophysiology of blepharospasm and oromandibular dystonia. *Brain* 1985;**108**:593–608.
6 Elston JS. A new variant of blepharospasm. *J Neurol Neurosurg Psychiatry* 1992;**55**:369–71.
7 Elston JS. Long term results of treatment of idiopathic blepharospasm with botulinum toxin injections *Br J Ophthalmol* 1987;**71**(9):664–8.
8 Elston JS, Marsden CD, Grandas F, Quinn NP. The significance of ophthalmological symptoms in idiopathic blepharospasm. *Eye* 1988; 2:435–9.

9 Nielsen VK. Pathophysiology of hemifacial spasm: a reversible pathophysiologic state. *Neurology* 1984;**34**:418–26.

10 Leporr F. Bilateral cerebral ptosis. *Neurology* 1987;**37**:1043–6.

11 Goldstein JE, Cogan DG. Apraxia of lid opening. *Arch Ophthalmol* 1965;**73**:155–9.

Index

Page numbers in **bold** refer to figures; those in *italic* to tables or boxed material.

magnetic resonance angiography
40–2, **43**, 63, 99
magnetic resonance imaging
36–40, 99
magnocellular cells 2, 13
Marcus Gunn phenomenon 137,
206
Marcus Gunn pupil 185
medulloblastoma 131
Meige's syndrome 194, 200
melanin, anterior visual pathway
development 11–12
melanoma, choroidal 37
melanoma–associated retinopathy
48
meningioma 194
chiasmal 204
hyperostosis 38, 40
in neurofibromatosis 2, 54
optic nerve 35, 91–3
imaging 39
parasellar 104
meningitis 113, 130
Mestinon *see* pyridostigmine
methanol toxicity 27, 96
methylprednisolone, giant cell
arteritis 66
methylprednisolone 177
Meyer's loop 14, 109
migraine *174*, 175–6
acephalgic 176
childhood ophthalmoplegic 141
Millard–Gubler syndrome 127,
197
Miller–Fisher syndrome 142, *143*
mitochondrial cytopathies
bilateral visual cortex disease
113
chronic progressive external
ophthalmoplegia 119–20
and dietary deficiency 96
Lebers hereditary optic
neuropathy 82–3, **84**
ptosis 205–6
retinopathy 46, 47, **49**
Möbius syndrome 127–8, 197
mononeuritis multiplex 66
mononucleosis, infectious 87, 198
morning glory disc 79

motion blindness, cerebral 2, 115
MRA *see* magnetic resonance
angiography
MRI *see* magnetic resonance
imaging
mucormycosis, orbito–cerebral
142
Müller cells 3, 32
Müller's muscles 195–6, 207
multiple evanescent white dot
syndrome *48*
multiple sclerosis
fluorescein angiography 29
and Lebers hereditary optic
neuropathy 82
and optic neuritis 86
pendular nystagmus 167–8
pupils 186
and retrobulbar neuritis 176–7
saccadic abnormalities 169
mumps, measles, rubella (MMR)
vaccine 87
myasthenia gravis 121–4, 134,
206
clinical features 122–3
facial palsy 198
investigations 123–4
myasthenic syndromes 124–5
pathogenesis 122
treatment 124
myelination, visual pathway
development 11
myokymia
facial 204
superior oblique 170
myopathy, ocular *see* ocular
myopathies
myotonic dystrophy 121, 198
ptosis 206
pupils 186
retinal degeneration *47*

nasopharyngeal carcinoma 143
neostigmine 124
neuroblastoma 191
neurodegenerative disease
occipital cortex 113
retinal involvement 46–8